## EDITORS

**John D. Fernstrom, Ph.D.** is Professor of Psychiatry, Pharmacology, and Behavioral Neuroscience at the University of Pittsburgh School of Medicine, and Director, Basic Neuroendocrinology Program, Western Psychiatric Institute and Clinic.

Dr. Fernstrom graduated in 1969 from the Massachusetts Institute of Technology (MIT), Cambridge, Massachusetts, with a B.S. degree in Biology, and obtained his Ph.D. degree in Nutritional Biochemistry in 1972, also from MIT. He was a post-doctoral fellow in neuroendocrinology at the Roche Institute for Molecular Biology (Nutley, New Jersey). Before coming to the University of Pittsburgh, Dr. Fernstrom was an Assistant and then Associate Professor in the Department of Nutrition and Food Science at MIT.

Dr. Fernstrom has served on numerous governmental advisory committees, and is presently a member of the National Advisory Council of the Monell Chemical Senses Center, and is chairman of the Neuroscience Section of the American Institute of Nutrition. He is a member of numerous professional societies, including the American Institute of Nutrition, the American Society for Clinical Nutrition, the American Physiological Society, the American Society for Pharmacology and Experimental Therapeutics, the American Society for Neurochemistry, the Society for Neuroscience, and the Endocrine Society.

Among other awards, Dr. Fernstrom received the Mead-Johnson Award of the American Institute of Nutrition, a Research Scientist Award from the National Institute of Mental Health, a Wellcome Visiting Professorship in the Basic Medical Sciences, and an Alfred P. Sloan Fellowship in Neurochemistry.

Dr. Fernstrom has presented over 100 invited lectures and seminars at universities, and at national and international meetings. He has published over 150 research and review articles. His current major research interest concerns the influence of the diet and drugs on the synthesis of neurotransmitters in the central and peripheral nervous systems.

**Gregory D. Miller, Ph.D.** is Vice President of Nutrition Research/Technical Services for National Dairy Council® (NDC), Rosemont, Illinois.

Dr. Miller graduated in 1978 from Michigan State University with a B.S. degree in Nutrition and in 1982 earned an M.S. degree in Nutrition (Toxicology) from Pennsylvania State University. In 1986 he received a Ph.D. in Nutrition (Toxicology) from Pennsylvania State University.

He served as an Undergraduate Research Assistant in Nutrition-Toxicology at Michigan State University in 1978 and was a Graduate Research Assistant in the Center for Air Environment Studies and Nutrition Department of Pennsylvania State University from 1979 to 1986. Dr. Miller was a Research Scientist for Kraft, Inc., Glenview, Illinois from 1986 to 1989 and was a Senior Research Scientist from 1989 to 1992.

Dr. Miller is a member of the Society for Investigative Nutrition, the American College of Nutrition and the American Institute of Nutrition. He is a scientific advisory panel member for the Office of Technology Assessment for the development of a report on issues in the treatment and prevention of osteoporosis. He has chaired or co-chaired more than 10 workshops and symposia for national organizations including the Federation of American Societies for Experimental Biology and the International Life Sciences Institute – Nutrition Foundation.

Among other awards, he has received the 1989 Kraft Basic Science Award and was listed in the 1992 American Men and Women of Science and the 1992 Who's Who in Science.

Dr. Miller has presented more than 25 invited lectures at national and international meetings and has published more than 35 research papers, reviews, and abstracts. He has co-edited 2 books on diet and nutrition and contributed chapters to 4 books.

# Introduction to Book

**John D. Fernstrom and Gregory D. Miller**

The momentum for this volume derives from a recent meeting on the influence of nutrition on the central nervous system (Nutrition and Central Nervous System Function), organized under the auspices of the *Keystone Conferences* and sponsored by the *International Life Sciences Institute*. One of the principal topics of this meeting was the influence of dietary macronutrients on appetite regulation, and the impact of macronutrient substitutes on this relationship. In the course of the meeting, it became apparent that a considerable body of information concerning this issue had recently been developed. Moreover, many new ideas evolved from the discussion, suggesting that this research focus was generating considerable interest and activity in the scientific community. This recognition led us to consider the timeliness of a book covering this area of research, both from the standpoint of summarizing a new and developing body of knowledge, and from the viewpoint that a presentation of this information, in one place, might help stimulate thought and activity in this discipline. Accordingly, we have organized a set of articles that deals with several aspects of the issue of caloric and macronutrient intake regulation, and the impact of macronutrient substitutes on this relationship.

The book has been organized into three sections. The first presents two perspectives on appetite regulation in children and adults. Birch and Johnson (Chapter 1) discuss from a behavioral approach the development of food intake regulatory mechanisms in infants, from the nursing period when they appear mainly responsive to caloric cues, into childhood as they develop the appetite customs of their cultures. They present data showing that children, but not adults, have the ability to compensate calorically from meal-to-meal, and to balance total caloric intake over the 24-h period. However, by preschool age, they observe that individual differences in compensating ability appear, and argue from their data that some of these differences follow from cues regarding food intake acquired from their social environment (e.g., from parent eating habits and child-rearing strategies). Bray (Chapter 2) discusses the regulation of energy balance and food intake in adults from a more mechanistic viewpoint, and highlights potential sites of malfunction in a putative system for regulating caloric balance that might permit imbalance and thus lead to obesity. These articles convey the impression that while recent information offers new insights into caloric regulation, much work remains to be done before a sufficient understanding of the behavioral, metabolic, and physiologic features of food intake and caloric regulation emerges to allow for fully effective strategies to be developed for treating individuals with weight and appetite problems.

The second section takes as a point of departure the overview provided by Bray, and discusses in more detail some of the chemical and neural mechanisms possibly involved in appetite regulation and caloric homeostasis. Teff (Chapter 3) discusses the cephalic phase reflexes. These are neurally-mediated metabolic reflexes involving the brain that are initiated by the orosensory stimulation of food prior to digestion and absorption. She focuses on cephalic phase insulin secretion, and considers the roles it might play in hunger and in glucose homeostasis, and how abnormal cephalic phase insulin release might contribute to the development of diabetes and obesity. Fernstrom (Chapter 4) discusses evidence regarding a postprandial chemical/metabolic mechanism by which meal ingestion might inform the brain regarding macronutrient ingestion (and thus possibly influence subsequent appetite): meal-induced changes in the plasma amino acid pattern that rapidly alter the brain uptake of L-tryptophan and its conversion to the neurotransmitter serotonin. Available evidence indicates that the brain might sense the recent ingestion of protein and carbohydrate by such a mechanism, but not fat. Friedman and Rawson (Chapter 5) focus on a different chemical mechanism potentially linking food intake, metabolism, and subsequent appetite. They present data suggesting that food ingestion and other metabolic phenomenon influence hepatic ATP production by inducing changes in hepatic carbohydrate and fat oxidation, and thereby lead to an alteration in afferent vagus traffic to the brain that modifies appetite. This model seeks to identify a common metabolic mechanism, in this case located in the periphery, through which total caloric intake can be monitored by the brain, rather than the ingestion of any particular macronutrient. Finally, Ritter and Calingasan (Chapter 6) provide a somewhat different view on the monitoring of carbohydrate and fat utilization, offering evidence that while fatty acid utilization is monitored in the periphery, glucose metabolism is sensed directly in the brain. They suggest that this division of energy substrate sensing is consistent with the known primacy of glucose as an energy substrate for brain, in contrast to the widespread use peripherally of fatty acids as an energy source.

The third section focuses principally on caloric balance and the effects that macronutrient substitutes have on caloric intake and body weight. Caloric and noncaloric sweeteners are considered first. Schiffman et al. (Chapter 7) discuss the innate preference for sweet taste in humans (and other animals), and how it is influenced by state of nutriture and age. They further consider the influence of sweet taste on hunger and food intake, and argue that sweet taste per se does not generally stimulate appetite. Accordingly, they conclude that the use of noncaloric sweeteners in the diet does not produce an unwanted stimulation of food intake. However, Blundell and Rogers (Chapter 8) also examine the influence of sweet taste on appetite and arrive at a different conclusion, based on their reading of available data, viz., that sweetness *does* stimulate appetite, or rather that sweetness weakens the satiating effect of food (calories). Finally, Black and Anderson (Chapter 9) provide a third perspective on this issue. They argue from population data on sugar consumption over the past half-century that sweetness in the diet does not correlate with the incidence of obesity, and thus that dietary sweetness appears not to be linked to excessive calorie intake. Further, regarding nonnutritive sweeteners, they note that the ability of such agents to reduce long-term caloric intake is not yet proven, and thus that their utility in long-term weight control is presently unclear.

The dietary preference for fat, fat ingestion, and the use of fat substitutes to reduce caloric intake are then considered in several articles. Drewnowski (Chapter 10) discusses the importance of the sensory properties of food to selection. He notes that in general, sweet and fat tastes are hedonically favored, with the *combination* of both tastes in foods being most favored. He argues that while carbohydrate "craving" has been argued to be the cause of overeating in the obese, recent data suggest that the common dietary feature among obese subjects is an expressed preference for *fat*, not carbohydrate. Harris (Chapter 11) presents findings from dietary fat studies in rats. Her results indicate that the animals do not compensate calorically when excessive fat is added to the diet, and show increases in fat deposition and body weight. Reducing the fat content of the diet reversed these effects, either by substituting carbohydrate or fat-mimetics. Harris concludes that palatable foods containing fat substitutes may be useful in promoting a reduction in fat intake by the general population. Rolls and Shide (Chapter 12) discuss results in humans showing that normal-weight males that are unrestrained eaters appear to detect the caloric density of foods (where fat content has been covertly manipulated to alter caloric density), and adjust intake to maintain constancy of caloric intake. Compensation is not achieved, however, by modifying fat intake. In contrast, restrained eaters appear to detect only poorly the caloric density (fat content) of food, suggesting they may be vulnerable to overeating fat. Levitsky and Strupp (Chapter 13) examine the influence of chronic changes in dietary fat content on caloric intake and body weight in women who are slightly overweight. Reducing dietary fat content reduced caloric intake and body weight, with the subjects compensating only gradually for the reduced caloric content of the foods over the 11-week period. And despite ultimate caloric compensation, the loss of body weight was maintained. The findings suggest that reducing dietary fat intake may be an effective way to reduce body weight. Rolls and Shide, and Levitsky and Strupp thus appear to differ in their conclusions regarding the potential utility of low-fat foods for reducing caloric intake and body weight. However, too few studies have been performed to date on this issue to allow a firm conclusion. This recognition will hopefully stimulate further work on this topic.

Finally, Levine and Billington (Chapter 14) discuss the use of dietary fiber as a potential method for reducing caloric intake and body weight. From the available data, they argue that if an effect is present, it is modest, and conclude that dietary fiber is probably not efficacious as a method for controlling body weight and appetite.

Overall, the articles in this book provide a glimpse into a developing area of investigation. They show a portion of the ongoing effort to determine if and how humans regulate their intake of nutrients, as well as some of the potential mechanisms by which such regulation may be affected, and consider whether macronutrient substitutes for carbohydrate and fat may be usefully applied to help control caloric intake and body weight. We hope that the assembly of this information in one volume will serve as a platform to highlight this area of investigation, as well as to stimulate future research.

University of Pittsburgh
Pittsburgh, Pennsylvania
and
National Dairy Council
Rosemont, Illinois

## CONTRIBUTORS


**G. Harvey Anderson, Ph.D.**
Department of Nutritional Sciences
Faculty of Medicine
University of Toronto
Toronto, Ontario, Canada

**Charles J. Billington, M.D.**
Department of Food Science and Nutrition
University of Minnesota
Minneapolis, Minnesota

**Leann L. Birch, Ph.D.**
Department of Human Development and Family Studies
College of Health and Human Development
The Pennsylvania State University
University Park, Pennsylvania

**Richard M. Black, Ph.D.**
Department of Nutritional Sciences
Faculty of Medicine
University of Toronto
Toronto, Ontario, Canada

**John E. Blundell, Ph.D.**
Biopsychology Group
Psychology Department
University of Leeds
Leeds, United Kingdom

**George A. Bray, M.D.**
Pennington Biomedical Research Center
Louisiana State University
Baton Rouge, Louisiana

**Noel Y. Calingasan, D.V.M., Ph.D.**
Burke Rehabilitation Center
Cornell University Medical College
White Plains, New York

**Adam Drewnowski, Ph.D.**
Human Nutrition Program
School of Public Health
University of Michigan
Ann Arbor, Michigan

**John D. Fernstrom, Ph.D.**
Department of Psychiatry, Pharmacology, and Behavioral Neuroscience
University of Pittsburgh School of Medicine
Pittsburgh, Pennsylvania

**Mark I. Friedman, Ph.D.**
Monell Chemical Senses Center
Philadelphia, Pennsylvania

**Ruth B. S. Harris, Ph.D.**
Nutrition Department
Kraft General Foods, Inc.
Glenview, Illinois

**Susan L. Johnson, Ph.D.**
Department of Human Development and Family Studies
The Pennsylvania State University
University Park, Pennsylvania

**Allen S. Levine, Ph.D.**
Research Services
VA Medical Center
Minneapolis, Minnesota

**David A. Levitsky, Ph.D.**
Division of Nutritional Sciences
Cornell University
Ithaca, New York

**Maureen Mackey, Ph.D.**
The NutraSweet Company
Deerfield, Illinois

**Gregory Miller, Ph.D.**
Nutrition Research/Technical Services
National Dairy Council
Rosemont, Illinois

**Nancy E. Rawson, Ph.D.**
Monell Chemical Senses Center
Philadelphia, Pennsylvania

**Sue Ritter, Ph.D.**
Department of Veterinary and Comparative Anatomy, Pharmacology, and Physiology
College of Veterinary Medicine
Washington State University
Pullman, Washington

**Peter J. Rogers, Ph.D.**
Consumer Sciences Department
Agricultural and Food Research Council
Institute of Food Research
Reading Laboratory
Reading, United Kingdom

**Barbara J. Rolls, Ph.D.**
Program in Behavioral Health
College of Health and Human Development
The Pennsylvania State University
University Park, Pennsylvania

**Susan S. Schiffman, Ph.D.**
Departments of Psychiatry and Psychology: Experimental
Duke University
Durham, North Carolina

**David J. Shide, Ph.D.**
Program in Behavioral Health
College of Health and Human Development
The Pennsylvania State University
University Park, Pennsylvania

**Barbara J. Strupp, Ph.D.**
Division of Nutritional Sciences and
Department of Psychology
Cornell University
Ithaca, New York

**Karen Teff, Ph.D.**
Monell Chemical Senses Center
Philadelphia, Pennsylvania

**Zoe S. Warwick, Ph.D.**
Departments of Psychiatry and Psychology: Experimental
Duke University
Durham, North Carolina

## TABLE OF CONTENTS

## Section III
## MACRONUTRIENT INTAKE, CALORIC COMPENSATION, AND THE IMPACT OF MACRONUTRIENT SUBSTITUTES

# *I. Evidence for Regulation and Caloric Sensitivity*

# Introduction

**G. Harvey Anderson**

Many factors are involved in the central nervous system's regulation of appetite. To rationalize all of the putative factors found to play a role, several integrative models have been proposed. One of these models, as proposed by Bray, is described in Chapter 2 and attests to a current view of the physiologic and metabolic factors that may be involved and how they interact in an integrated system. This model assumes that in adults food intake and energy balance are determined primarily by internal control mechanisms. A contrasting view is presented in Chapter 1 by Birch and Johnson. They suggest that in children internal systems can operate relatively precisely to maintain energy intake on a daily basis, although there is great individual variation on a meal to meal basis. However, the internal control can be completely overridden by external factors, particularly parental control. Implicit in their discussion is the suggestion that eventually some individuals adapt to regulate caloric intake only by external cues. These are not new points of view. However, common to both chapters is the hypothesis that it is some characteristic of food, related to its macronutrient composition or to its hedonic properties that accounts for energy imbalance. The latter has received frequent analysis in the past. The former has become of greater interest in the past 20 years, beginning with evidence that experimental animals could quantitatively control their intake of macronutrients and that some control systems were present for this purpose. Errors in these control systems, particularly in those responding to carbohydrate intake, have been offered as an explanation for the development of certain human eating disorders.[1]

The role of diet composition in determining energy imbalance remains unclear, however. For many years, added sugar was blamed for causing gluttony. It was assumed that its sweet taste encouraged overeating because the sensory stimulus overrode any caloric signals arising from its metabolic utilization. Yet a look at consumption of sugar over the past 50 years provides little evidence of an association with the increased prevalence of obesity in the North American population.[2] Although high-intensity sweeteners were developed on the premise that the population would be healthier if sweetness was consumed separately from calories, their widespread usage for the past decade has done little to curb the increasing incidence of obesity. A more current hypothesis is that fat is the culprit. Increased availability and consumption of fat does tend to associate with the increase in incidence of obesity. Furthermore, there are experimental data showing that (1) fat is stored with greater metabolic efficiency than carbohydrate; (2) if diets are equal calorically, higher body weights are maintained when the diet is high in fat than when it is high in carbohydrate; and (3) children do not adjust caloric intake in a subsequent meal if the test meal is high in fat rather than high in carbohydrate (Birch and Johnson, Chapter 1).

If fat is the culprit, then it is worth wondering if the availability of high intensity sweeteners has been counterproductive to the dietary goals of reducing fat intake. When sugar is consumed sweetness is derived from carbohydrate calories. If a high-intensity sweetener is consumed, it is most often associated with essentially no calories, leaving a caloric deficit that may be replaced by fat calories.[3] In contrast, reducing fat calories by replacing them with carbohydrate or with fat substitutes offers the potential for reducing fat and energy intake by both replacement of fat in a food and by shifting energy replacement to carbohydrate.[3] Nevertheless, it should be borne in mind that the human has a readily adaptable metabolic capacity, and that obesity occurs in populations consuming diets of high fat or high carbohydrate composition. Thus, at present, there is little evidence to suggest that a change in dietary macronutrient composition, at least to the extent recommended by current dietary guidelines, will offer the solution to the high incidence of obesity in the North American population.

As indicated in the two chapters that follow, the evolutionary process has generated a complex regulatory system that remains a puzzle. Indeed, given the complexity attributed to the regulatory system and its seemingly endless list of control systems and signals, one can only be amazed that in most animals and humans it works as effectively as it does.

## REFERENCES


1. Anderson, G. H., Black, R. M., and Li, E. T. S. Physiological determination of food selection: association with protein and carbohydrate. In: *Feast and Famine: Relevance to Eating Disorders,* G. H. Anderson and S. Kennedy, Eds. New York, Academic Press, 1991, 73.
2. Anderson, G. H. Sugar consumption: are dietary guidelines needed?, *J. Can. Diet. Assoc.,* 50, 229, 1989.
3. Beaton, G. H., Tarusak, V., and Anderson, G. H. Estimation of possible impact of non-caloric fat and carbohydrate intake in the human, *Appetite,* 19, 87, 1992.

# 1 Appetite Control in Children

**Leann L. Birch and Susan L. Johnson**

The selection of an adequate variety and quantity of food is crucial to children's growth and health. From a developmental perspective, during the early years of life, the child must negotiate a transition from suckling to feeding, which involves a dramatic change in what is consumed and in the extent to which the child controls the feeding process. Initially, the young infant depends on a single food source, so that food selection is not an issue. The infant is probably the only depletion driven human eater; even in the first weeks of life, there is evidence that infants are responsive to depletion cues. For example, infants adjust the volume of a feeding in response to (1) alterations in the energy density of milk, consuming larger volumes of less energy dense preparations[1,2] and (2) variations in intermeal intervals, such that larger feedings are taken following longer intervals.[3]

As development proceeds, children must begin to adopt the adult diet of the culture, and they acquire food preferences, which become major determinants of food selection. Appetite comes increasingly under the control of experiential, sociocultural, and cognitive factors. Children are learning what to eat, when to eat, even how much to eat, and which foods are appropriate to the context. These factors interact with genetic predispositions to produce increasing diversity in how individuals control food intake and how successfully they maintain energy balance. It is our working hypothesis that individual differences in styles of intake control can be conceptualized as differences among individuals' responsiveness to physiological feedback and to sociocultural and to cognitive factors in controlling their food intake. With the many opportunities we have for eating, the relative salience of these factors continues to be shaped by individual experience, so that by adulthood, styles of intake control have been acquired that differ markedly across individuals.

Although it is generally agreed that individual differences in styles of intake control exist among adults, there is currently no consensus regarding how they should be measured and characterized. However, there is evidence that adults differ in the extent to which they continue to be responsive to

0-8493-4466-2/94/$0.00+$.50

energy density of foods in adjusting their food intake in response to covert manipulations of the energy density of foods.[4-7] Furthermore, individual differences in the extent to which adults succeed in maintaining a stable desirable weight are obvious, and even among those who maintain their weight, differences exist in the extent to which this maintenance is achieved effortlessly or only through strategies such as calorie counting and dietary restraint. Characterizing the precise nature of such individual differences among adults is beyond the scope of this chapter, although it is our hope that this review will shed more light on the possible etiology of such differences. This chapter will focus on the role of energy density in appetite control during early childhood, and on some of the factors that influence the extent to which children's intake is controlled by responsiveness to energy density. The first portion of the chapter reviews the initial evidence that in an experimental protocol children can adjust their intake in response to covert manipulation of the energy density of foods. In subsequent sections of the chapter we will explore the more complex questions of whether such short-term adjustments within single meals are consistent with the evidence regarding the adjustments in total daily energy intake seen under free living conditions, and under what conditions these adjustments in intake occur. Finally, some evidence will be reviewed that suggests familial factors are centrally important in the etiology of individual differences in the controls of food intake.

## I. RESPONSIVENESS TO ENERGY DENSITY: SINGLE MEAL PROTOCOLS

In a series of experiments conducted in our laboratory, we have investigated children's responsiveness to energy density in controlling their food intake.[8-10] In these experiments, children consumed fixed amounts of one food as a first course preload, followed after a short delay by a second eating occasion. The first meal consisted of a single food that can vary in energy density, based on manipulating the carbohydrate or, more recently, the fat content of that food, while keeping the sensory characteristics as similar as possible. The second meal consisted of a variety of foods, selected to vary in macronutrient content, and sensory characteristics. The delay between the first and second meals has varied from about 5 min to 1 h, but has typically been 15 or 20 min. On some days, children consumed the high-energy density version, on others the low energy density version. The children's *ad libitum* consumption of the second self-selected meal following the different preloads provided the data on the question of interest: Do children adjust their energy intake in response to the energy density of the first course preload?

Results of these experiments indicate that children are responsive to energy density, eating more following the low- than the high-energy density preloads. The adjustment in intake typically occurs on the first opportunity; repeated experience with the preloads is not necessary to see the subsequent adjustment in intake, at least when the energy density of the preloads is altered by varying their carbohydrate content. In one experiment, we compared the intake patterns of children with those of a group of adults.[9] Subjects consumed the high or low-energy density preloads before a self-selected lunch, on separate days 1 week apart. Children showed clear evidence of caloric compensation; as a group, the children reduced their intake following the high energy preload by about 110 kcal, the difference in the energy content of the preloads. In contrast, the adults showed no clear evidence for such adjustment in subsequent intake; they ate nearly identical lunches following the two preloads. The data also provide evidence that the adult sample was much more variable than the children with respect to whether they adjusted their intake in response to the energy density of the preload: only 60% of adults consumed more following the low- than the high-energy density preload; 95% children showed this pattern of intake, although there were individual differences among children in how precisely they compensated for the energy in the preloads.

Subsequent experiments have corroborated the basic finding that children can adjust their intake in response to the energy density of the preload, and that this is the case regardless of whether the time delay between the two eating occasions is 5 min or 1 h. More recently, we have investigated whether children show such adjustments in subsequent intake when energy density is manipulated by altering the fat content of preloads.[11] Although our data are limited, the results suggest that adjustments in subsequent intake in response to fat manipulations are less precise and develop more slowly than those described in response to carbohydrate manipulations. In the experiments involving manipulations of fat content, children were given repeated opportunities to consume the preloads, and to eat a subsequent meal *ad libitum*. In contrast to the immediate adjustments in intake when carbohydrate content of the preloads is manipulated to alter energy density, clear evidence for responsiveness to the manipulation of dietary fat content of the preloads appeared only after the children had repeated opportunities to eat the preloads. We will return to this difference in responsiveness to energy from fat vs. carbohydrate in the next section, which discusses the evidence for children's regulation of energy intake over 24-h periods.

We have also analyzed the patterns of *ad libitum* consumption to determine how these relatively precise adjustments in intake are accomplished.[12] One possibility we explored was that the children's energy compensation was also macronutrient specific. Such macronutrient specific compensation would require that, following a high-fat, high-energy preload, children would select food to produce low-fat meals. The data have provided no evidence for such macronutrient-specific compensation. A second possibility is that children were selecting the same foods following the high- and low-energy preloads, but their compensation resulted from their consuming smaller amounts of all the same foods following the high-energy preloads. The data were not consistent with this hypothesis. However, when we examined the children's *ad libitum* intake based on their preferences for the foods served *ad libitum,* we found that they were continuing to consume similar amounts of their most preferred foods across the preload conditions, but as energy density increased, consumption of nonpreferred foods was suppressed.[13]

In a related set of experiments designed to explore conditioned satiety and conditioned preferences, children were given repeated opportunities to consume preloads varying in energy density, and in which a flavor cue was always paired with the same energy density. In this case, after repeated trials, children adjust their intake in a subsequent meal by learning to associate a distinctive flavor cue with the energy density of the food.[8] This provides a possible mechanism for children to learn to anticipate the feelings of satiety provided by foods differing in energy density, and adjust subsequent intake accordingly. Children who have had repeated experience with consuming distinctively flavored preloads that also differ in energy density learn to prefer the flavor paired with high energy density, and this effect is potentiated by hunger.[14] In both these protocols, in which children have the opportunity to repeatedly consume the preloads, followed by the *ad libitum* meals, we see especially clear evidence for individual differences among children in the accuracy with which they adjust their subsequent intake. This accuracy is listed as a percentage, with 100% indicating that *ad libitum* intake was reduced by exactly the amount of energy in the preload, and 0% indicating no adjustment in intake in response to the differences across the preloads. As already indicated, children reduce their intake following the high-energy preload, but there are individual differences in how precisely they compensated: some children showed no compensation at all while others compensated for 100% of the preload calories.[8] Individual differences in the extent to which children are responsive to energy density in adjusting their intake are already apparent by the preschool period.

We have begun to explore the possibility that differences in child feeding practices could be contributing to individual differences in children's responsiveness to energy density cues.[15] Children participated in a series of conditioning trials that took place in one of two child feeding contexts. One was designed to mimic a context in which the adults attempted to externally control the child's eating: children were told it was time to eat, and were focused on the amount of food remaining on the plate and were rewarded for eating. In contrast, in the other context, the adults discussed feelings of hunger and satiety with the children, and had discussions regarding how these feelings should be used to decide when to eat, how much to eat, and when to stop eating. Results indicated that with the imposition of external controls, responsiveness to energy density disappeared, and children showed no compensation in response to preload energy density. However, children in the "internal" condition responded in a manner similar to children seen in the previous experiments and adjusted their intake in response to the energy density of the preloads. This experimental evidence suggests that child feeding practices, especially the extent to which parents impose external controls on children's eating, may be a crucial factor in producing individual differences in children's responsiveness to energy density. However, producing such effects in the laboratory says little about the extent to which they arise as a result of family interactions that occur in the feeding context.

## II. RESPONSIVENESS TO ENERGY DENSITY: EVIDENCE FOR REGULATION OF 24 H ENERGY INTAKE

The research described above has been limited to a very short time frame: children's ability to adjust energy intake in response to alterations in the energy density within the same meal, or within an hour or so. We have also been investigating the extent to which children show adjustments in energy intake over 24-h periods, which allows us to look for adjustments in energy intake across successive meals[16,17] and to look for individual differences in how accurately children adjusted their energy intake. In this research, we measured the intake of 2- to 5-year-old children on all six eating occasions each day, over a series of days (6 days in one case, 8 days in the other). The research was conducted in the naturalistic context of the children's normal daycare and home settings. Two measures that we obtained are particularly relevant to the issue of individual differences in children's ability to adjust intake. These measures were possible because we had obtained the first measured intake data on young children's food intake over a series of days. First, we were able to calculate coefficients of variation (CVs) for each child for each of the six meals consumed each day (breakfast, morning snack, lunch, afternoon snack, dinner, and evening snack), and for total daily energy intake. Second, we calculated correlations on the children's energy intake across successive meal pairs for individual children. This latter measure allowed us to look at the extent to which children were adjusting their intake across successive meals, for example, by taking a large breakfast and following it with a small snack. Because there were six meals eaten each day, there were five successive meal pairs, and five correlations were calculated for each child. Negative correlations provided evidence for meal-to-meal compensation in intake. We simply used the number of negative correlations (from 0 to 5) for each child as an index of meal-to-meal compensation in energy intake.

Examination of the CVs for energy intake at meals and for total daily energy intake revealed that across all children, the variability of individual meals was very high, and much greater than the variability of total daily energy intake. While CVs for individual meals were on average, about 30%, CVs for total daily energy intake were only about 10%. The majority of the correlations between energy intake at one meal and the next were negative, providing evidence for meal-to-meal compensation in energy intake.

The CVs for each individual child for the six meals and for total daily energy intake are depicted in Figure 1. Each child is represented as a data point at each meal and for total daily energy intake. As is very evident in the figure, individual differences in these CVs were very large. We hypothesized that the pattern of large CVs for meals relative to the low CV for total daily energy intake was being produced by compensatory intake across meals. If this were the case, then children with the smallest CVs for total daily energy intake should show the strongest evidence of compensation in energy intake across successive meals. When we correlated each child's CV for total daily energy intake with that child's compensation index (the number of negative correlations in energy intake across successive meals), we found that the two measures were significantly negatively correlated in both experiments, ($r = -0.51$, $p < 0.05$) as we hypothesized. Total daily energy intake was relatively tightly regulated and this was accomplished, at least in part, by compensation in energy intake across successive meals. In these more naturalistic contexts, children also provided clear evidence that they were adjusting their energy intake across meals to maintain a relatively constant total energy intake over 24-h periods. There were clear individual differences in how successfully children were able to do this. The question that remains is whether these individual differences can be related to differences in the children's experiential history or to familial variables.

## III. RESPONSIVENESS TO ENERGY DENSITY: INDIVIDUAL DIFFERENCES IN RELATION TO FAMILIAL ANTHROPOMETRICS AND FEEDING PATTERNS

We have recently obtained evidence suggesting that individual differences among children's responsiveness to energy density is related to the style of parenting adopted by mothers and fathers, and, in particular, how

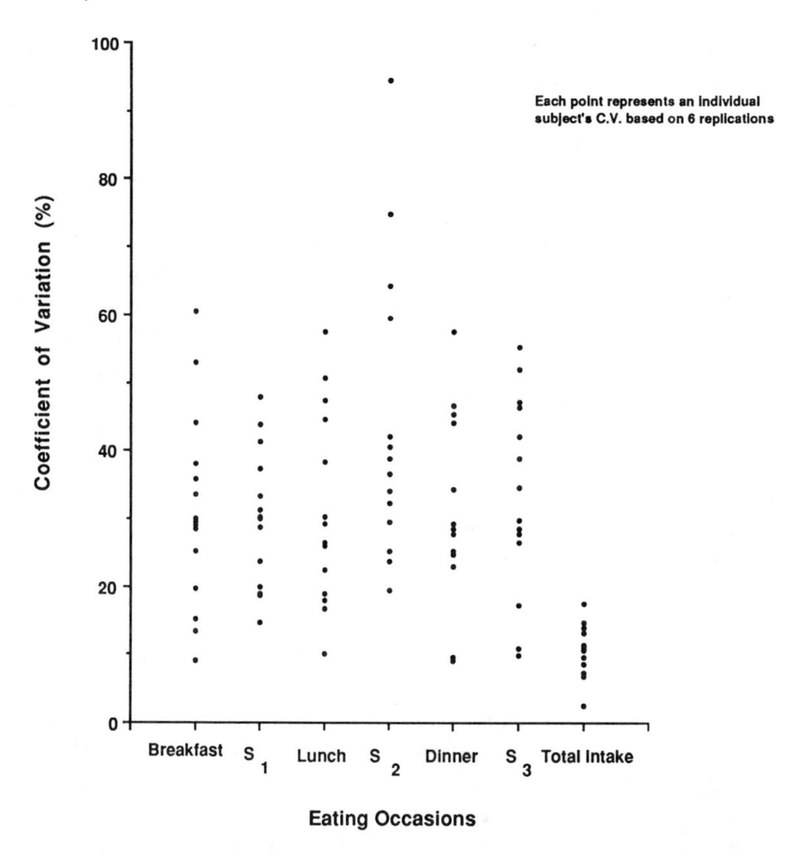


**FIGURE 1.** Coefficients of variation (CVs) for energy intake at meals and for total daily energy intake; $S_{1,2,3}$ = morning, afternoon, and evening snack, respectively.[16]

authoritarian parents are. Costanzo and colleagues' ideas on obesity proneness and domain-specific parenting[18] suggest that parents apply especially rigid external controls over their children's behavior in domains in which (1) the child is potentially deviant, (2) the parents are particularly concerned or invested, and (3) they do not believe the child can acquire the necessary skills on their own. In the case of obesity proneness, parents who are overweight and who struggle unsuccessfully with their own weight would be expected to impose a great deal of external control on their children's eating: they see the child as potentially deviant, are concerned about the child becoming obese, and in that they, as parents, cannot successfully control their own food intake, they do not believe the child can either. Therefore, the imposition of authoritarian, external controls of feeding should impede the development of children's internal controls. We have begun to explore the extent to which such relationships exist between parental practices and weight status and our measure of children's internal control in the feeding context: the degree to which children are responsive to energy density in controlling their food intake.

Using the Parent Attitude Research Instrument (PARI-Q4 and PARI[19,20]) as a global measure of parenting style, we correlated parents' self reports of authoritarianism with children's compensation patterns during a single meal protocol. We found a negative relationship ($r = -0.27$, $p < 0.08$) between parents' degree of authoritarianism and children's percentage compensation for preload calories: parents who were more authoritarian had children who were less responsive to energy density in controlling their food intake.[21] Consistent with other research on the relationship between parenting style and various child outcomes, including self-reliance, problem solving, and social agency,[22] the negative relationship between authoritarianism and the degree of compensation was especially strong in boys ($r = -0.58, p < 0.008$). This suggests that boys may be particularly susceptible to control strategies used in the home environment. Further research studying the impact of parents' child feeding strategies on children's compensation patterns should employ a more domain-specific assessment of the degree of control exerted by parents over the child's eating behaviors.

Children's responsiveness to energy density is also related to parent adiposity and dieting history. Parents were asked to report their height and weight and to complete the Three Factor Eating Questionnaire (TFEQ[23]). The TFEQ measures three aspects of eating style: (1) dietary restraint, (2) disinhibition, or the loss of restraint, and (3) perceived hunger. We hypothesized that parents who employed a large degree of cognitive control in managing their own diet would be likely to impose external controls upon their children's eating behaviors, and, by extension, these children would show less evidence of compensation during single meal protocols.

Parental body mass indices (BMI) were calculated and correlated to scores for each factor of the TFEQ and to children's compensation patterns. Significant relationships were found between (1) parent anthropometric measures and TFEQ scores and (2) children's compensation patterns and parent questionnaire and anthropometric data. Parent BMI was strongly positively correlated, not to restraint, but to parents' reports of disinhibition ($r = 0.69, p < 0.0001$). In our sample, the heavier adults were those who have difficulty in *stopping* eating once they start, as opposed to highly restrained individuals having any particular success or failure at dieting. Furthermore, father's BMI was negatively correlated to children's percentage compensation ($r = -0.31$, $p < 0.02$): heavier fathers have children who are less responsive to energy density. When analyzed by gender, only girls' compensation patterns were related to father's BMI ($r = -0.43$, $p < 0.03$). Mother's BMI did not significantly correlate to either boys or girls eating patterns. Finally, parents' disinhibition scores were negatively correlated with children's percentage compensation ($r = -0.29$, $p < 0.04$), suggesting that parents' disinhibited eating may be providing a model for their children's eating behaviors.

These preliminary findings suggest that the home environment, in particular parent eating patterns and child-rearing strategies, are potentially powerful influences on the development of children's eating styles. Although the impact of these parental variables on children's adiposity is yet to be determined, the data suggest how the social environment could contribute to well-documented familial patterns of obesity.

## CONCLUSION

In controlling their food intake, children are generally responsive to energy density cues, and this leads to adjustments in intake, such that they tend to consume a larger meal following a smaller first course. Observation of children's energy intake over 24-h periods reveals that compensation also occurs across successive meals, so that relatively large meals are followed by relatively small ones. This pattern of meal-to-meal compensation gives rise to a pattern of energy intake that is highly variable at meals, while for 24-h periods, energy intake is relatively consistent.

Data from both single meal protocols and from 24-h energy intake reveal differences among children in the extent to which they are controlling intake in response to energy density. The initial evidence suggests that this individual variation in the development of internal controls of food intake are related to parental eating patterns, adiposity, and child-rearing strategies.

## REFERENCES

1. Fomon, S. J., Voluntary food intake and its regulation. In *Infant Nutrition*, 2nd ed., W. B. Saunders, Philadelphia, 1974, 20.
2. Allen, J. C., Keller, R. P., Archer, P., and Neville, M. C., Studies in human lactation: milk composition and daily secretion rates of macronutrients in the first year of lactation, *Am. J. Clin. Nutr.*, 54, 69, 1991.
3. Matheny, R., Birch, L. L., and Picciano, M. F., Control of intake by human milk fed infants: relationships between feeding size and interval, *Dev. Psychobiol.*, 23, 511, 1990.
4. Rolls, B. J., Pirraglia, P., Jones, M., and Peters, J., Effect of covert fat replacement with olestra on 24-hour food intake in lean adults, *Fed. Am. Soc. Exp. Biol.*, 5, 4100A, 1991.
5. Mattes, R. D., Pierce, C. B., and Friedman, M. I., Daily caloric intake of normal-weight adults: response to changes in dietary energy density of a luncheon meal, *Am. J. Clin. Nutr.*, 48, 214, 1988.

6. Foltin, R. W., Fischman, N. W., Moran, T. H., Rolls, B. J., and Kelly, T. H., Caloric compensation for lunches varying in fat and carbohydrate content by humans in a residential laboratory, *Am. J. Clin. Nutr.,* 52, 969, 1990.
7. Lissner, L., Levitsky, D. A., Strupp, B. J., Kalkwarf, H. J., and Roe, D. A., Dietary fat and the regulation of energy intake in human subjects, *Am. J. Clin. Nutr.,* 46, 886, 1987.
8. Birch, L. L., McPhee, L., Steinberg, L., and Sullivan, S., Conditioned flavor preferences in young children, *Physiol. Behav.,* 47, 501, 1990.
9. Birch, L. L., and Deysher, M., Caloric compensation and sensory specific satiety: evidence for self regulation of food intake by young children, *Appetite,* 7, 323, 1986.
10. Birch, L. L., and Deysher, Conditioned and unconditioned caloric compensation: Evidence for self-regulation of food intake by young children, *Learn. Motiv.,* 16, 341, 1986.
11. Johnson, S. L., McPhee, L., and Birch, L. L., Conditioned preferences: young children prefer flavors associated with high dietary fat, *Physiol. Behav.,* 50, 1245, 1991.
12. Birch, L. L., Bryant, J., McPhee, L., and Johnson, S. L., Children's lunch intake: effects of midmorning snacks varying in energy density and fat content, *Appetite,* 20, 83, 1993.
13. Birch, L. L., McPhee, L., and Sullivan, S., Children's food intake following drinks sweetened with sucrose or aspartame: time course effects, *Physiol. Behav.,* 45, 387, 1989.
14. Kern, D. L., McPhee, L., Fisher, J., Johnson, S. L., and Birch, L. L., The postingestive consequences of fat condition preferences for flavors associated with high dietary fat, *Physiol. Behav.,* 54, 71, 1993.
15. Birch, L. L., Shoba, B. C., Steinberg, L., and Krehbiel, R., "Clean up your plate": effects of child feeding practices on the conditioning of meal size, *Learn. Motiv.,* 18, 301, 1987.
16. Birch, L. L., Johnson, S. L., Andresen, G., Peters, J. C., and Schulte, M. C., The variability of young children's energy intake, *N. Engl. J .Med.,* 324, 232, 1991.
17. Birch, L. L., Johnson, S. L., Jones, M. B., and Peters, J. C., Effects of Olestra, a non-caloric fat substitute, on children's energy and macronutrient intake, *Am. J. Clin. Nutr.,* (1993) In press.
18. Costanzo, P. R., and Woody, E. Z., Domain-specific parenting styles and their impact on the child's development of particular deviance: the example of obesity proneness, *J. Soc. Clin. Psychol.,* 3, 425, 1985.
19. Schludermann, S., and Schludermann, E., A methodological study of a revised maternal attitude instrument: Mother's Pari Q4, *J. Psychol.,* 95, 77, 1977.
20. Schludermann, S., and Schludermann, E., Response set analysis of a paternal attitude research instrument (Pari), *J. Psychol.,* 79, 213, 1971.

21. Johnson, S. L., and Birch, L. L., Children's sensivity to energy density is related to parents' eating and disciplinary styles, *J. Cell. Biochem.,* 16B, WB104, 1992.
22. Baumrind, D., Current patterns of parental authority, *Dev. Psychol. Monograph,* 48, 1, 1971.
23. Stunkard, A. J., and Messick, S., The Three-Factor Eating Questionnaire to measure dietary restraint, disinhibition, and hunger, *J. Psychosom. Res.,* 29, 71, 1985.

# 2 Appetite Control in Adults

**George A. Bray**

There are several approaches to understanding appetite and food regulation in adults. There are behavioral models, metabolic models, and set-point models that can be used. This chapter will present a nutrient balance or homeostatic model for the control of nutrient stores.[1] Obesity and anorexia nervosa can be viewed as a homeostatic failure of nutrient balance resulting from a failure of nutrient signals to be properly integrated into an effective feedback system. It is hoped that this approach will provide a useful system for understanding appetite control and obesity.

## I. THE NUTRIENT BALANCE OR HOMEOSTATIC MODEL

A regulated, homeostatic or controlled system has several components (Figure 1). First, there is a controller located in the brain. Second, there is a control system consisting of intake, digestion, absorption, storage, and metabolism of the nutrients in food. Third, there are feedback elements that tell the controller about the state of the controlled system. Finally, there are the efferent control mechanisms that modulate food intake and energy expenditure.

## II. THE CONTROLLED SYSTEM

The normal adult human being contains approximately 140,000 kcal of energy in body fat. This is some six times the quantity of energy that is stored in protein (24,000 kcal). By comparison, the quantity of carbohydrate is minute, equivalent to only 800 kcal, which includes glycogen stores from liver, kidney, muscle, and other tissues plus the glucose that circulates in the blood. An individual eating 2000 kcal of which 40% is carbohydrate will take in an amount of carbohydrate each day comparable to their total body stores. In contrast, average daily protein intake is only a little over 1% of total stores and fat intake considerably less than 1%. This relationship of storage pool size to daily intake for each

0-8493-4466-2/94/$0.00+$.50

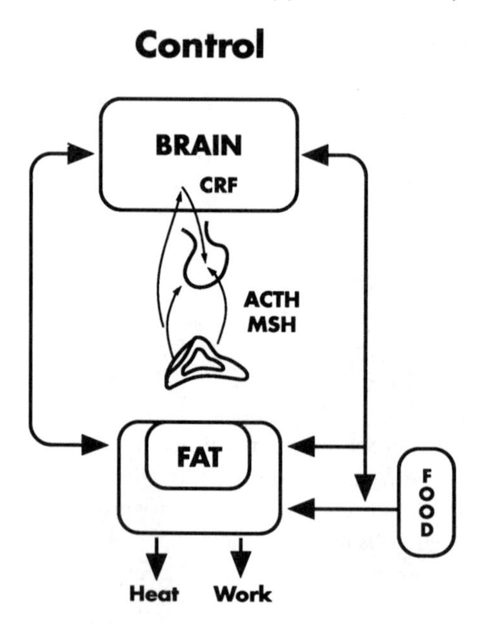


**FIGURE 1.** Diagram of a controlled system. The controller for food intake is located in the brain, which received afferent signals from the periphery and integrates them into efferent controls that produce food intake and modulation of the controlled system of nutrient intake storage and oxidation. (Copyright 1989, George A. Bray. Used with permission.)

macronutrient is depicted in Figure 2. From the figure it becomes clear why Flatt has argued from studies in animals that changes in carbohydrate balance affect carbohydrate intake reciprocally and rapidly from day to day, whereas changes in fat balance do not seem to affect fat intake appreciably.[2]

There are two major pathways for absorption of digested food from the gut. One of these pathways is through the lacteals, which transport triglycerides packaged as chylomicrons. These enter the venous circulation and are cleared in the periphery by hydrolysis of triglycerides catalyzed by the enzyme lipoprotein lipase. The other pathway for absorption of glucose and amino acids as well as short-chain fatty acids is through the portal vein directly to the liver. The nutrients that enter the controlled system can be stored, converted to heat through metabolism, or used for work. In addition, small quantities can be excreted in the urine as the end-products of amino acid metabolism.

The resting metabolism of human beings is directly related to the amount of fat free or lean body mass.[3] In addition, there is an important familial component in energy expenditure.[4] Physical work accounts for approximately ⅓ of the energy expended. That body weight and energy stores are well

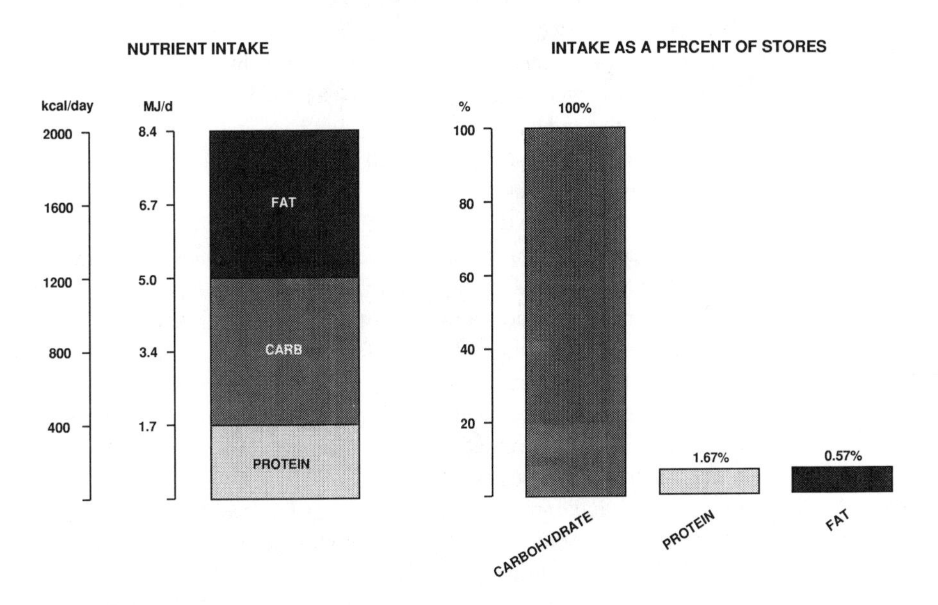


**FIGURE 2.** Relationship of nutrient intake to body stores. A diet containing 40% fat, 40% carbohydrate, and 20% protein is shown on the left in terms of energy. The relationship of each of these components to the body stores of the corresponding nutrient is shown on the left side as a percent of nutrient stores. (Copyright 1989, George A. Bray. Used with permission.)

regulated over short intervals in most individuals has been suggested in a number of studies. For most adults the sensitivity of the system for changes is less than 1% per year.[5]

An analysis of this regulatory control system suggests the following concepts:

1. That each major nutrient is regulated separately and then integrated into total energy needs.
2. That the time required to achieve balance for each nutrient varies as a function of the amount ingested each day in relation to the total body

stores of that nutrient. Thus becoming obese by eating a high carbohydrate diet would appear to be more difficult than with a high-fat diet because the body storage system for carbohydrate as glycogen is limited. This is shown most convincingly in data from Brazil.[6] The weight of subgroups within the population rose as the percent of calories from dietary fat increased. Similarly, after World War II the migration of individuals from Japan, where lower fat diets are the norm, to Hawaii or North America, where high-fat diets are the norm was associated with an increase in the prevalence of obesity in these individuals. Although excess carbohydrate can be converted to fatty acids, this is an energetically expensive transformation. Body fat stores, on the other hand, are many times larger than daily fat intake implying a much greater capacity for fat storage and a much longer time constant to achieve balance.

3. Achievement of nutrient balance requires that the net oxidation of each nutrient equals the average composition of the macronutrients in the diet. That is, ingestion of a high-fat diet requires greater oxidation of fat than a low-fat diet when equilibrium is achieved.
4. There are major differences between individuals in the capacity to increase rapidly the oxidation of fat after beginning a high-fat diet. Much of this difference is genetic.
5. Physical training can increase oxidation of fatty acids by muscle and thus regular aerobic exercise might reduce the tendency to become obese when eating a high-fat diet.
6. The regulation of nutrient stores is subject to positive and negative feedback signals for each component that operate through the central controller.

Composition of the diet plays a variable role in the development of obesity in man and animals. At one extreme are the types of obesity depicted in stone age carvings.[7] Obesity in these women developed regardless of the type of diet available. In these instances, genetic factors probably play an important role since experimental animals with genetically transmitted obesity become obese no matter what type of diet. At the other extreme are those types of obesity where dietary composition is central to the development of obesity. These include a high-fat diet, and diets with an abundance of highly palatable foods. Any of these dietary obesities can be controlled by changing diets along with restraint in levels of food intake.

## III. AFFERENT FEEDBACK SIGNALS

The brain receives information for regulating nutrient balance from several sources. Afferent signals can be transmitted over the somatic sensory nervous system from visual, auditory, or other signals, via the autonomic nervous system or through the blood stream from internal information.

### A. Sensory Signals

The sight and smell of food are important signals for identifying potential sources of food and initiating food intake. Along with the texture and taste of food in the mouth, the sensory cues about the quality of food can serve as either positive feedback signals for initiating or continuing food ingestion or negative feedback signals that eventually slow down, terminate, or abort an eating incident. The ability of animals to avoid foods that have previously made them sick, a phenomenon known as bait-shyness, is an example of these afferent sensory signals integrated with a central learning system.

### B. Gastrointestinal Signals

Information from food in the gastrointestinal tract can be initiated by one of three mechanisms. The first is gastrointestinal distension, the second is release of gastrointestinal hormones when nutrients act directly on the gastrointestinal tract, and the third is through the effects of absorbed nutrients.

Pharyngeal, esophageal, gastric, and intestinal distension may all be mechanisms for terminating meals by negative feedback via the nervous system. The vagus nerve is probably the principal afferent sensory relay for these types of information.

Several gastrointestinal hormones have been implicated in the inhibition of feeding. The one studied most intensively has been cholecystokinin (CCK).[8] Intraperitoneal injections of CCK decrease food intake in hungry rats as well as inhibiting sham feeding in rats and monkeys. Sham feeding in these experiments is giving liquid diets to animals with drainage cannulas in the stomach or esophagus so that food is drained out before it can enter the intestine. Furthermore, the sequence of events associated with a response to CCK is similar to that of spontaneous postprandial satiety. One suggestion for the effect of CCK is that it acts on antral CCK (CCK-A) receptors by constricting the pylorus and enhancing gastric distension. Peripheral information generated by CCK may be important in producing satiety since vagotomy will block the effect of CCK. In clinical studies, CCK-8 (the sulfated octapeptide fragment from CCK) inhibits food intake as effectively in patients with hypothalamic injury, which produces obesity as in obese controls.[9]

A second site of action for CCK could be within the central nervous system itself. CCK is released in the brain during a meal and the injection of CCK into the ventromedial hypothalamus has been reported to reduce food intake and increase sympathetic activity. Thus CCK might act on the CCK-B receptors specific to this area, but most studies suggest that the

CCK-B receptors in the brain are less important than the CCK-A receptors in the gut in producing satiety to CCK. Other peptides such as bombesin[10] and the N-terminal pentapeptide from procolipase[11] may also be signals produced in the gastrointestinal tract that inhibit feeding.

### C. Nutrient Signals

Nutrient signals may also act on the liver or brain to initiate satiety. Either glucose or arginine injected into the portal circulation decreases the vagal afferent firing rate probably by acting on hepatic glucose receptors. Glucose may also act directly on the central nervous system since this nutrient is the major source of fuel for the brain. Hauger et al. demonstrated that glucose regulates the binding of amphetamine to the sodium pump in the hypothalamus and that this effect is modulated by the intake of glucose.[12] Moreover, analogs of glucose that block glucose metabolism will increase food intake probably by acting on medullary hindbrain gluco–receptors.[13]

Fatty acids and their metabolites may also serve as afferent signals to modulate food intake. Injection of either 3-hydroxybutyrate or lactate produces satiety.[14] Conversely, blockade of fatty acid oxidation increases feeding.[15]

Lactate is a potentially interesting metabolite for modulation of food intake. Injections of lactate, such as 3-hydroxybutyrate, decrease food intake. Lactate is produced in adipose tissue, muscle, and other tissues by metabolism of glucose. It is a primary end-product during glucose metabolism by fat cells and might serve as a metabolic signal from this tissue. Tumors frequently produce a decrease in food intake and weight loss. Tumors may also produce considerable amounts of lactate, which might be anorectic. Finally, metformin and phenformin, two oral agents for treatment of diabetes, increase lactate levels. When compared to sulfonylurea-like drugs, phenformin was more effective at reducing body weight. This might be related to its effect on lactate production. The hypothesis that lactate is an afferent signal for satiety requires more testing.

## IV. THE CONTROLLER

### A. Anatomy

Several anatomic regions of the brain appear to play an important role in the control of nutrient balance. Destruction of the ventromedial hypothalamus (VMN) is associated with hyperphagia and obesity in most homeothermic species that have been studied.[16] On the other hand, destruction of the lateral hypothalamus is associated with a decrease in food intake and a reduction in body fat. More recently, the paraventricular

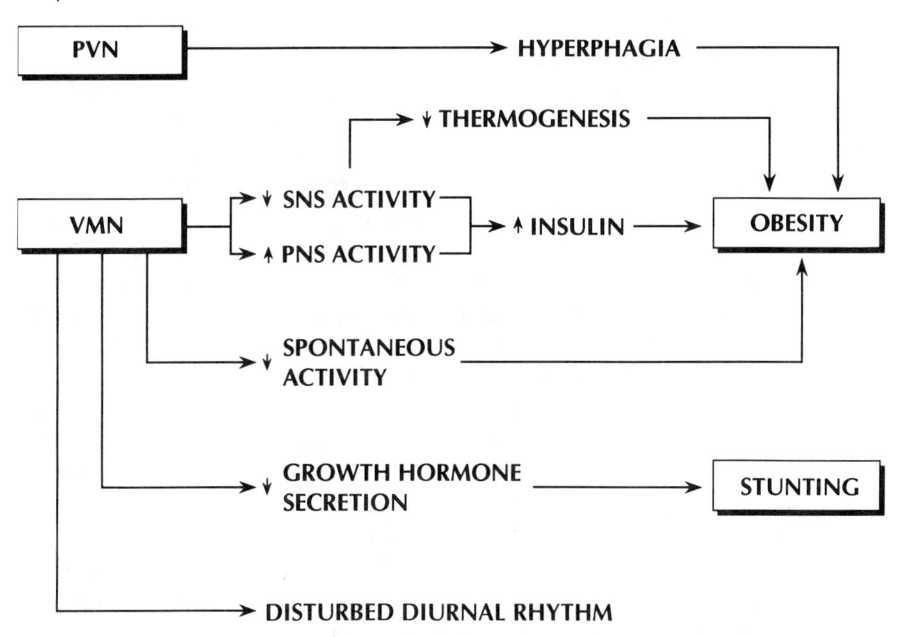


**FIGURE 3.** Comparison of the effects of PVN and VMN lesions. PVN lesions produce hyperphagia, which is a sine qua non for development of obesity. A VMN produces an imbalance in the function of the autonomic nervous system and a decrease in growth hormone and activity. (Copyright 1991, George A. Bray. Used with permission.)

nucleus (PVN) has been shown to be a particularly important region for stimulation of food intake following topical injection of norepinephrine, which acts through $\alpha_2$-adrenergic receptors.[17] Figure 3 shows a model for the effects of PVN and VMN lesions. Damage to the PVN produces hyperphagia, which appears to be necessary and sufficient to produce obesity. In contrast, a VMN lesion can produce obesity regardless of whether hyperphagia develops. While the VMN lesion produces multiple physiologic effects, the decrease in sympathetic activity and increase in parasympathetic activity (the autonomic hypothesis) appear to be essential for the development of obesity.[16]

## B. Neurotransmitters

### 1. Amino Acids Neurotransmitters

Four amino acids are found in high concentration in the brain. Glutamate and aspartate stimulate neuronal discharge whereas γ-aminobutyric acid (GABA) and glycine inhibit neuronal activity. γ-Aminobutyric acid is the only amino acid neurotransmitter involved in the regulation of food intake.[18] It can either stimulate or inhibit feeding depending on where it is acting.

### 2. Monoamine Neurotransmitters

There are a number of monoamine neurotransmitters that modulate feeding, including norepinephrine, serotonin, and histamine. The monoamines act more slowly, i.e., have a longer latency than amino acid neurotransmitters. The concentration of the monoamine neurotransmitters in brain is 0.1 to 1.0% that of the amino acids. These monoamines appear to act through surface receptors on intracellular second messengers within neurons. Serotonin is derived from the dietary amino acid tryptophan. This neurotransmitter reduces food intake. Norepinephrine can decrease food intake by activating β receptors in the perifornical area or stimulate food intake by acting on $\alpha_2$-adrenergic receptors in the paraventricular or ventromedial nucleus.[17] A comparison of the tonic level of adrenergic receptor activation in the hypothalamus of genetically obese and lean animals showed that in the lean rats, the tonic activity of β-adrenergic receptors was higher and the tonic activity of $\alpha_2$-adrenergic receptors was lower than in the obese animal. Thus a shift in the tonic activity from β to $\alpha_2$ receptors is associated with obesity. Histamine is the third monoamine that affects food intake. Activation of H-1 histamine receptors reduces food intake in the ventromedial hypothalamus.[19]

### 3. Peptidergic Neurotransmitters

Several peptides also modulate food intake[16,20] as shown in Table 1. The concentration of these peptides in brain is about 0.1 to 1% that of the monoamines (pg/g vs. ng/g). Neuropeptide Y, β-endorphin, dynorphin, growth-hormone-releasing hormone, and galanin all stimulate food intake when injected into the third ventricle, or into the ventromedial or paraventricular nucleus. A variety of other peptides including bombesin, cholecystokinin, enterostatin, anorectin, calcitonin, neurotensin, and corticotropin-releasing hormone inhibit feeding when injected into either the third ventricle or the ventromedial nucleus.

One hypothesis to explain the role of neuropeptides in modulation of food intake is through their effects on specific types of eating.[1,21] This is summarized in Table 2. Thus neuropeptide Y injected into the paraventricular nucleus preferentially increases carbohydrate intake and galanin increases fat intake.[22] Enterostatin, vasopressin, and corticotropin-releasing hormone inhibit fat intake.[21] The infusion of insulin into the third ventricle will suppress food intake in animals eating a high carbohydrate diet but not in animals eating a low carbohydrate (high-fat) diet.[23] These examples suggest that the way in which these peptides act is to modulate the intake of specific nutrients as part of the homeostatic system dealing with individual "appetites". This nutrient-specific hypothesis can explain the concept of sensory specific satiety.[24] This hypothesis proposes that the preference for food

**TABLE 1**
**Peptides That Stimulate or Suppress Feeding**

| Increase food intake | Decrease food intake |
|---|---|
| Dynorphin | Anorectin (CTPG) |
| β-Endorphin | Calcitonin (CGRP) |
| Galanin | Cholecystokinin (CCK) |
| Growth hormone-releasing hormone (GHRH) | Corticotropin-releasing hormone (CRH) |
| Neuropeptide Y (NPY) | Cyclo-His-Pro |
| | Enterostatin (VPDPR) |
| | Glucagon |
| | Insulin |
| | Neurotensin |
| | Oxytocin |
| | Vasopressin |

decreases relative to other foods after a preferred food has been eaten. The ability to modulate specific nutrient intake can easily provide a mechanism for changing the preference to specific foods.

## V. EFFERENT CONTROLS

The efferent controls include the motor activities involved in identifying, obtaining, and ingesting food as well as the efferent effects produced by the

**TABLE 2**
**Peptides Affecting Specific Nutrients**

| Nutrient | Increase | Decrease |
|---|---|---|
| Fat | Galanin<br>Opioids<br>β-Casomorphin | Enterostatin<br>Vasopressin<br>Corticotropin-releasing hormone |
| Carbohydrate | Neuropeptide Y<br>Insulin | Cholecystokinin |
| Protein | Growth hormone-releasing hormone | Glucagon |
| Sodium | Angiotensin | |

autonomic nervous system and several circulating hormones. The complex sequence of motor activities that leads to the initiation of food seeking, the identification of food, and the killing and ingestion of this food is integrated in the lateral hypothalamus, since electrical stimulation in this area will lead to food seeking and ingestive behavior.[16] Further discussion of this system is beyond the scope of this review. The other components are discussed below.

## A. Autonomic Nervous System

### 1. Parasympathetic Nervous System

Both the sympathetic and parasympathetic nervous systems may be involved in the development of obesity. In animals where obesity follows hypothalamic lesions there is evidence for increased activity of the efferent parasympathetic nervous system (vagus nerve). This provides part of the explanation of the increase in insulin secretion that characterizes this syndrome.[16]

### 2. Sympathetic Nervous System

Reduction in sympathetic activity is also characteristic of the obese state and may participate in the enhanced insulin secretion.[25] In the experimental animal there is an inverse relationship between the activity of the sympathetic nervous system and food intake.[25,26] In spontaneously feeding rats there is a negative correlation throughout the 24 h between basal activity of the sympathetic nervous system and spontaneous food intake. In addition almost all of the experimental maneuvers we have tested that increase food intake, such as lesions in the ventromedial hypothalamus or genetic obesity, decrease the activity of the sympathetic nervous system.[25] Conversely, those maneuvers that decrease food intake, such as lateral hypothalamic lesions or injections of fenfluramine, an appetite suppressant drug, increase sympathetic activity. These reciprocal relationships are shown in Table 3.

The nature of the reciprocal relationship can be viewed as follows. The afferent relays in the vagal complex in the medulla connect to the perifornical feeding system, which has an efferent input into the vagal and sympathetic complex in the medulla. Hypothalamic efferent sympathetic fibers also provide input into the vagal complex on their way to the periphery. Thus any sympathetic efferent activity could modulate afferent signals, which modulate hypothalamic feeding through an inhibitory pathway from the medullary vagal complex. These possibilities and the effects of peptides on the sympathetic nervous system are shown in Figure 4.

**TABLE 3**
**Relationship of Food Intake and Sympathetic Activity**

| Experimental procedure | Lesion or injection site | Effect of treatment on: Food intake | SNS[1] activity |
|---|---|---|---|
| Lesion | PVN | ↑ | → |
| Lesion | VMH | ↑ | ↓ |
| Lesion | LH | ↓ | ↑ |
| Norepinephrine | VMH | ↑ | ↓ |
| Serotonin | VMH | ↓ | ↑ |
| Neuropeptide Y | PVN | ↑ | ↓ |
| β-Endorphin | 3rd ventricle | ↑ | ↓ |
| CRH | 3rd ventricle | ↓ | ↑ |
| Cholecystokinin | 3rd ventricle | ↓ | ↑ |
| Anorectin | 3rd ventricle | ↓ | ↑ |
| 2-Deoxy-D-glucose | i.c.v. | ↑ | ↓ |
| Fenfluramine | i.p. | ↓ | ↑ |
| Nicotine | s.c. | ± | ↑ |
| Mazindol | i.p. | ↓ | ↑ |
| *d*-Amphetamine | i.p. | ↓ | ↑ |
| Diethylpropion | i.p. | ↓ | → |

## B. Efferent Hormonal Mechanisms

### 1. Insulin

Increased levels of insulin are characteristic of obesity. Injections of insulin can increase food intake and produce obesity, probably by lowering glucose concentrations. Injections of 2-deoxy-D-glucose, an analog of glucose, stimulates food intake by inhibiting intracellular glucose metabolism and producing glucoprivation. Insulin has been proposed as a signal to the brain about the quantity of peripheral fat stores. One major problem with this hypothesis is that insulin levels fall rapidly following caloric restriction and long before there are any significant changes in the quantity of body fat. Moreover, there are some experimental types of obesity which occur with little or no rise in the concentration of insulin.[28]

There are two other interpretations of the hyperinsulinemia of obesity. First, the rise in insulin may be a reflection of high levels of nutrient intake. Since insulin is essential for nutrient storage increased flux of nutrients would be expected to increase insulin. Second, hyperinsulinemia may reflect actual or apparent hypothalamic resistance to insulin action. In this case increased

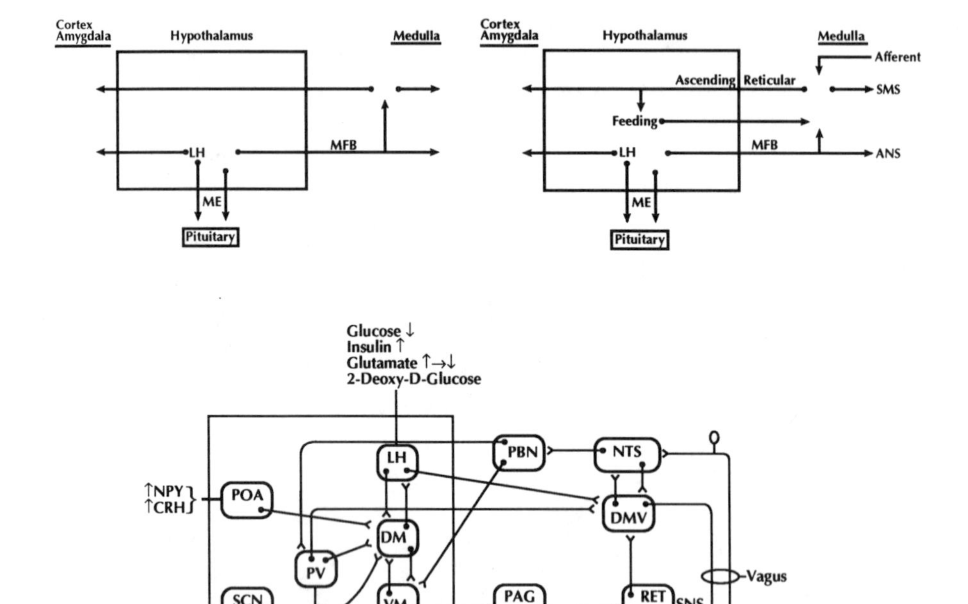


**FIGURE 4.** Model for the effects of peptides on food intake and the sympathetic nervous system. The diagram on the top left shows the functions of the hypothalamus, which are to control the pituitary secretions, send messages rostrally and caudally, and to route signals from the hindbrain rostelly. On the upper right center which received input from the ascending reticular pathways and sends signals to the hindbrain. Thus, any signal from the sympathetic tracts in the MFB could provide feedback messages to the feeding center and this in turn could modulate the hindbrain. The diagram to the bottom shows a number of hypothalamic and hindbrain nuclei and the peptides or nutrients that have been shown to modulate their activity. (Copyright 1991, George A. Bray. Used with permission.)

insulin secretion would be modulated by changes in the function of the autonomic nervous system resulting from resistance to the action of insulin in the central nervous system.

## 2. Adrenal Steroids

The development or progression of experimental obesity is either reversed or attenuated by adrenalectomy. In clinical medicine Addison's disease with adrenal insufficiency is associated with loss of body fat whereas Cushing's syndrome with high levels of adrenal steroid secretion is associated with obesity. The fact that almost all defects in genetically obese animals are reversed by adrenalectomy and that clinical change in adrenal status can produce leanness or obesity suggest that glucocorticoids play a key role in the development and maintenance of the obese state.[16,25,28] Obesity is a failure of this homeostatic model for nutrient balance. It appears to be a failure of nutrients to stimulate the sympathetic nervous system that requires permissive levels of adrenal glucocorticoids. The sympathetic nervous system may fail to be stimulated because afferent signals are not generated effectively or because the receptors for these signals in the central nervous system do not respond adequately or because the signals are not transduced into effective efferent messages. A recent model proposes that obesities represent increased sensitivity to glucocorticoids resulting from loss of a peptide that modulates steroid responsive genes.[29]

## VI. SUMMARY AND CONCLUSION

Obesity can be most easily conceptualized as a problem of defective control of normal feedback systems. This homeostatic approach is used as the basis for considering the relative importance of individual nutrients and other elements of the control system. The diet normally consists of about 50% carbohydrate, 35% fat, and 15% protein. Relative to body stores, the amount of carbohydrate eaten each day is similar to what is stored as glycogen, whereas the stores of fat and protein are greatly in excess of the daily intake. Studies with experimental animals suggest that the control of body fat content is more stable on a high carbohydrate diet than on a high-fat diet. Moreover, to maintain energy balance requires that the average daily intake of carbohydrate and fat must be the same as the mix of carbohydrate and fat that is used as fuel by the body. Regular physical exercise enhances the oxidation of fat and may thus play a role in maintaining lower body fat stores. Although increasing body fat is observed when most animals and probably humans eat a high-fat diet, this is not always the case. There must, therefore, be mechanisms by which the rate of fat oxidation can be increased in the face of a high-fat diet. Information about the intake of nutrients and about body nutrient stores is relayed to the brain by afferent signals. These signals can be the nutrients themselves, hormones released by interactions of nutrients with the gut, or by the effects of food and its nutrients on neural messages to the brain. From this wealth of afferent information the brain must sort out the relevant signals and make decisions about food intake. These processes are integrated in the hypothalamus, among other areas. Several neurotransmitters are involved in this intraneuronal signaling, including γ-aminobutyric acid, norepinephrine, serotonin, and several peptides. The various peptides used in this process may act to modulate specific types of food intake. Thus neuropeptide Y stimulates carbohydrate and galanin stimulates fat intake. Fat intake is reduced by enterostatin intake, corticotropin-releasing hormone, and CCK. Once the brain has made a decision, efferent processes are initiated. The animal or human can search for food, or stop eating. When food is ingested, the autonomic nervous system and endocrine system are involved in partitioning the ingested macronutrients into body stores. High levels of sympathetic activity are associated with lower levels of body fat. Absence of adrenal glucocorticoid hormones is also associated with lower levels of body fat. On the other hand, high levels of insulin are associated with higher levels of body fat. From this nutrient balance model, it is possible to understand the mechanisms involved in the control of appetite and in the development of obesity as well as approaches to its treatment.

## REFERENCES

1. Bray, G. A., Obesity — a disease of nutrient or energy balance, *Nutr. Rev.*, 45, 33, 1987.
2. Flatt, J. P., Assessment of daily and cumulative carbohydrate and fat balances in mice (technical note), *J. Nutr. Bioc.*, 2(4), 193, 1991.
3. Ravussin, E., Lillioja, S., Anderson, T. E., Christin, L., and Bogardus, C., Determinants of 24-hour energy expenditure in man: methods and results using a respiratory chamber, *J. Clin. Invest.*, 78, 566, 1986.
4. Bogardus, C., Lillioja, S., Ravussin, E., et al., Familial dependence of the resting metabolic rate, *N. Engl. J. Med.*, 315, 96, 1986.
5. Williamson, D. F., Kahn, H. S., Remington, P. L., and Anda, R. F., The 10-year incidence of overweight and major weight gain in U.S. adults, *Arch. Intern. Med.*, 150, 665, 1990.
6. World Health Organization. *Diet, Nutrition, and the Prevention of Chronic Diseases*, World Health Organization Technical Report Series, 1990, 797.
7. Bray, G. A., Obesity: historical development of scientific and cultural ideas, *Int. J. Obes.*, 14, 909, 1990.
8. Peikin, S. R., Role of cholecystokinin in the control of food intake, *Gastrointest. Endocrinol.*, 18, 757, 1989.
9. Boosalis, M. G., Gemayel, N., Lee, A., Bray, G. A., Laine, L., and Cohen, H., Cholecystokinin and satiety: effect of hypothalamic obesity and gastric bubble insertion, *Am. J. Physiol.*, 262, R241, 1992.
10. Gibbs, J., Fauser, D., Rowe, E., Rolls, B., Rolls, E., and Madison, S., Bombesin suppresses feeding in rats, *Nature (London)*, 282, 208, 1979.
11. Shargill, N. S., Tsujii, S., Bray, G. A., and Erlanson-Albertsson, C., Enterostatin suppresses food intake following injection into the third ventricle of rats, *Brain Res.*, 544, 137, 1991.

12. Hauger, R., Hulihan-Giblin, B., Angel, A., Luu, M., Janowsky, A., Skolnick, P., and Paul, S., Glucose regulates ($^3$H)(+)-amphetamine binding and Na+K+ATPase activity in the hypothalamus: a proposed mechanism for the glucostatic control of feeding and satiety, *Brain Res. Bull.,* 16, 281, 1986.
13. Ritter, R. C., Slusser, P. G., and Stone, S., Glucoreceptors controlling feeding and blood glucose: location in the hindbrain, *Science,* 213, 451, 1981.
14. Scharrer, E., and Langhans, W., Control of food intake by fatty acid oxidation, *Am. J. Physiol.,* 250, R1003, 1986.
15. Friedman, M. I., Body-fat and the metabolic control of food-intake, *Int. J. Obes.,* 14(S3), 53, 1990.
16. Bray, G., York, D., and Fisler, J., Experimental obesity: a homeostatic failure due to defective nutrient stimulation of the sympathetic nervous system, *Vit. Hormon.,* 45, 1, 1989.
17. Leibowitz, S. F., Brain monoamines and peptides: role in the control of eating behavior, *Fed. Proc. Fed. Am. Soc. Exp. Biol.,* 45, 1396, 1986.
18. Tsujii, S., and Bray, G. A., GABA-related feeding control in genetically obese rats, *Brain Res.,* 540, 48, 1991.
19. Sakata, T., Ookuma, K., Fukagawa, K., Fujimoto, K., Yoshimatsu, H., Shiraishi, T., and Wada, H., Blockade of the histamine $H_1$-receptor in the rat ventromedial hypothalamus and feeding elicitation, *Brain Res.,* 441, 403, 1988.
20. Morley, J., Neuropeptide regulation of appetite and weight, *Endocr. Rev.,* 8, 256, 1987.
21. Bray, G. A., Obesity — a disease of nutrient or energy balance?, *Nutr. Rev.,* 45(2), 33, 1987.
22. Leibowitz, S. F., Hypothalamic neuropeptide Y, galanin, and amines. Concepts of coexistence in relation to feeding behavior, *Ann. N.Y. Acad. Sci.,* 575, 221, 1989.
23. Arase, K., Fisler, J., Shargill, N., York, D., and Bray, G., Intracerebroventricular infusions of 3-hydroxybutyrate and insulin in a rat model of dietary obesity, *Am. J. Physiol.,* 255, R974, 1988.
24. Rolls, B. J., Sensory-specific satiety, *Nutr. Rev.,* 44, 93, 1986.
25. Bray, G. A., Obesity, a disorder of nutrient partitioning: the Mona Lisa Hypothesis, *J. Nutr.,* 121, 1146, 1991.
26. Sakaguchi, T., Takahashi, M., and Bray, G., Diurnal changes in sympathetic activity: relation to food intake and to insulin injected into the ventromedial or suprachiasmatic nucleus, *J. Clin. Invest.,* 32, 282, 1988.
27. Campfield, L. A., Brandon, P., and Smith, F. J., On-line continuous measurement of blood glucose and meal pattern in free-feeding rats: the role of glucose in meal initiation, *Brain Res. Bull.,* 14(6), 605, 1985.
28. Inoue, S., Animal models of obesity: hypothalamic lesions. In: *Obesity,* P. Bjorntorp, and B. Brodoff, Eds. J. B. Lippincott, Philadelphia, 1992, 266.
29. York, D. A., Genetic models of animal obesity. In: *Obesity,* P. Bjorntorp, and B. Brodoff, Eds. J. B. Lippincott, Philadelphia, 1992, 233.
30. Bray, G. A., York, D. A., Lavau, M., and Hainault, I., Adrenalectomy in the Zucker fatty rat: effect on m-RNA for malic enzyme and glyceraldehyde 3-phosphate dehydrogenase, *Intern. J. Obes.,* 15(10), 703, 1991.

# *II. Mechanisms of Caloric Compensation*

# Introduction

**John D. Fernstrom**

The chapters in this section focus on some of the putative mechanisms, currently under study, by which food affects brain circuits involved in metabolic and appetite regulation. The brain garners information regarding potential edibles at a variety of levels, which it uses to facilitate the ingestion, digestion, absorption, and distribution of nutrients within the body. This information enters the brain either in the process of food acquisition and ingestion, or after the food has been digested and absorbed into the circulation. As discussed by Teff, the information provided to the brain during food acquisition is acquired primarily via sensory receptors (vision, olfaction, taste), and input to the brain via afferent nerve fibers (optic, olfactory, autonomic). This information is believed to aid the brain, acting via efferent neural mechanisms, in optimizing food digestion and nutrient distribution. The information provided to the brain following food absorbtion is input via a multiplicity of mechanisms, some of which are discussed in the chapters by Fernstrom (Chapter 4), Friedman and Rawson (Chapter 5), and Ritter and Calingasan (Chapter 6). These mechanisms include the sensing of carbohydrate and fat fluxes in the body by the liver, and the provision of this information to the brain via afferent parasympathetic fibers, and the sensing of carbohydrate and amino acid (protein) fluxes directly within the brain. As should be apparent in reading these chapters, fairly convincing information is becoming available indicating that clear, metabolically-derived signals reach the brain that could be used to distinguish carbohydrate, fat, and protein utilization within the body. And some data suggest that food intake can be influenced by such signals. Nevertheless, it must also be noted that our knowledge in this area is rudimentary. Much further work will be necessary before we will have a useful understanding of the mechanisms by which the brain manages the metabolic economy of the body, and the use to which appetite and food intake are put as participants in this process.

# 3 Cephalic Phase Insulin Release in Humans: Mechanism and Function

**Karen Teff**

## I. CEPHALIC PHASE REFLEXES

Early in the twentieth century, Pavlov reported on what he termed "the psychic or appetite juices", physiological secretions elicited through cognitive and oral sensory stimulation.[1] In this series of classical experiments, animals were fitted with esophageal and gastric fistulas, allowing them to experience the olfactory and gustatory properties of the food, without the postabsorptive effects. Food was then inserted directly into the stomach and the degree of digestion evaluated, with and without oral stimulation. In this way, Pavlov clearly demonstrated the importance of sensory stimulation for salivary secretion and gastric acid release and for the optimization of digestion. Today, physiological responses released by oral sensory stimulation are usually referred to as cephalic phase reflexes.

Cephalic phase reflexes are rapidly occurring, autonomic and endocrine responses triggered by food-related sensory stimulation.[2] Stimulation of sensory receptors in the head and throat region send afferent signals to specific areas in the central nervous system, including the nucleus of the solitary tract.[3] Information is then relayed to the dorsal motor nucleus of the vagus, which sends parasympathetically-mediated vagal efferents to gastrointestinal tissues causing the release of compounds such as insulin, glucagon, gastric acid, and pancreatic exocrine enzymes.

Animal research has identified some of the sensory stimuli capable of eliciting the cephalic phase reflexes and their potential physiological function. However, relatively little is known about these reflexes in humans and not all findings from the animal literature can be extrapolated to man. In humans, most cephalic phase research has examined salivary secretion and gastric acid release with respect to sensory stimuli,[4] palatability,[5] and to

0-8493-4466-2/94/$0.00+$.50

some extent, physiological significance.[6] These studies have suggested that taste and palatability play an important role in eliciting the secretion of gastric acid and saliva.

## II. CEPHALIC PHASE INSULIN RELEASE

### A. Definition and Characterization

Cephalic phase insulin release (CPIR) has been demonstrated in a number of species including rat, dog, sheep, and man. In humans, there are less than 20 studies reported over the past 15 years (Tables 1 and 2).[7-23] Figure 1 illustrates a typical mean profile of CPIR from 15 normal weight subjects. In our laboratory, increases in insulin are observed by 2 min after sensory stimulation with a maximum peak occurring at 4 min poststimulus. Plasma insulin levels return to baseline between 8 and 12 min poststimulus. The magnitude of the increase is generally small relative to postprandial insulin release (7 to 30% above baseline), although there is a large interindividual variability with some subjects exhibiting rises of 100% above baseline. A number of laboratories[10,19,22,23] have reported that approximately 10 to 15% of both normal weight and obese subjects do not exhibit CPIR and therefore, could be classified as "nonresponders" (Figure 2). The lack of response may merely be a reflection of normal variation in insulin release or may be due to cognitive factors that have the potential to influence CPIR. Although there is some evidence of an association between an individual's attitude to food[18,22] and the magnitude of CPIR, psychological testing has not revealed a relationship between any particular psychological attribute and the absence of the response.

### B. Sensory Stimuli

To some extent, the observed variability in CPIR may be associated with differences in experimental design and methodology. As illustrated in Tables 1 and 2, different types of sensory stimuli ranging from hypnosis to visual and olfactory stimulation to actual ingestion of food have been used to elicit the response. The relative effectiveness of the different sensory stimuli have not been tested on CPIR, although work on gastric acid secretion suggests that increasing the complexity of the sensory stimulus, increases the magnitude of the response. For example, a modified sham feed in which subjects taste and chew food without swallowing was found to be the most effective stimulus for gastric acid release when compared to visual or olfactory stimulation alone.[4] With respect to CPIR, Bruce et al.[13] found that neither visual and olfactory stimulation nor sweet taste alone could stimulate CPIR, although in combination the two conditions were effective stimuli. Thus, the

**TABLE 1**
**Summary of Cephalic Phase Insulin Release (CPIR) Experiments in Normal Weight Subjects**

| Author | Date | Ref. | *n* (sex) | Stimulus | Conclusions |
|---|---|---|---|---|---|
| Goldfine et al. | 1970 | 7 | 7 (m/f) | Hypnosis | 3/7 subjects exhibit CPIR |
| Porte et al. | 1977 | 8 | 7 (m/f?) | Oral saccharin | Increase in insulin 20 min |
| Sahakian et al. | 1981 | 9 | 14 (m/f) | Visual/olfactory | CPIR |
| Bellisle et al. | 1983 | 10 | 7 (m/f) | Ingested sandwiches | CPIR |
| Bellisle et al. | 1985 | 11 | 10 (m/f) | Ingested sandwiches | CPIR |
| Yamazaki and Sakguchi | 1986 | 12 | 57 (m) | 0.5 ml glucose | CPIR |
| Bruce et al. | 1987 | 13 | 6 (m/f) | Visual/olfactory | No CPIR |
| | | | 5 (m) | Aspartame solution | No CPIR |
| | | | 7 (m) | Visual/olfactory + aspartame solution | CPIR |
| Lucas et al. | 1987 | 14 | 5 (m/f) | Savory tarts: whole and blended | Greater magnitude CPIR with whole food |
| Teff et al. | 1991 | 15 | 20 (m) | Ingested dessert | CPIR |
| Teff et al. | 1993 | 16 | 15 (m) | Sham-feed | CPIR |

closer the stimulus parallels actual food ingestion, the greater the cephalic phase response. With this hypothesis in mind, in our earlier experiments, we used a complex food system designed to maximize the elicitation of CPIR. The stimulus was a sweet, strawberry-flavored dessert primarily composed of dairy fat. This stimulus was not found to increase plasma glucose levels.[15,23] Subjects were permitted exactly 2 min to consume the food and the first blood sample collected immediately after the 2-min period. Other investigators have allowed subjects to consume food although the amount of food and the length of ingestion time were not controlled.[10,11,14] In these experiments, definition and verification of CPIR were dependent on a lack of increase in blood glucose during the early postingestive time period. However, although steady glucose levels support the assumption that increases in insulin are independent of glucose stimulation, the possibility still exists that there may be undetectable increases in blood glucose or other macronutrients such as protein[10,11] or fat[15] contained in the food are eliciting insulin release.

The experimental paradigm that allows maximal sensory stimulation without the possibility of a confounding postabsorptive effect is the modified sham-feed. Subjects are permitted to taste and chew the food but not

**TABLE 2**
**Summary of Cephalic Phase Insulin Release (CPIR) Experiments in Obese Subjects**

| Author | Date | Ref. | *n* (sex) | Stimulus | Conclusions |
|---|---|---|---|---|---|
| Parra-Covarrubias et al. | 1971 | 17 | 6 obese (m/f) | Visual/olfactory | CPIR |
| Rodin | 1978 | 18 | 3 obese (m/f?)<br>4 normal | Visual/olfactory | Increased CPIR in obese |
| | | | 11 obese<br>5 normal<br>5 formerly obese | Visual/olfactory | Graded CPIR response dependent on obesity and individual's response to external stimuli |
| Sjostrom et al. | 1980 | 19 | 25 obese (f)<br>23 normal (f) | Visual/olfactory | CPIR in obese<br>No CPIR in normals |
| Johnson and Wildman | 1983 | 20 | 4 obese (m/f)<br>6 normal (m/f) | Visual/olfactory | Increased CPIR in obese compared to normals |
| Osuna et al. | 1986 | 21 | 10 obese (f)<br>5 normal (m/f) | Visual/olfactory | CPIR in normals<br>No CPIR in obese |
| Simon et al. | 1986 | 22 | 15 obese (m/f)<br>10 normal (m/f) | Visual/olfactory | Increased CPIR in obese women |
| Teff et al. | 1993 | 23 | 15 obese (m)<br>18 normal (m) | Ingested dessert | No difference in magnitude of CPIR between obese/normal |

swallow it. This method of sensory stimulation was effective in eliciting salivary secretion and gastric acid release[4] but did not elicit an increase in plasma insulin.[24] In the latter experiment, blood sampling was not initiated until 5 min after stimulation and may have bypassed peak CPIR. We have recently used the modified sham-feeding paradigm with blood sampling beginning at 2 min postingestion and have found it effective in eliciting CPIR (Figure 1).[16] In fact, the modified sham-feed resulted in a CPIR profile identical to that observed after actual food ingestion. Visual and olfactory stimulation is another effective but slightly less complex sensory system that allows subjects to see and smell an appetizing meal but not taste it (Tables 1 and 2). Therefore, as in the modified sham-feed design, there is no postabsorptive effect. However, as there are some studies[13,19,21] in which visual and olfactory stimulation was not effective in eliciting CPIR, the lack of response may be due to inadequate sensory stimulation.

The simplest food-related sensory stimulus involves the administration of a single taste quality. In general, sweet has been the taste quality most often associated with eliciting CPIR. Animal research has repeatedly dem-

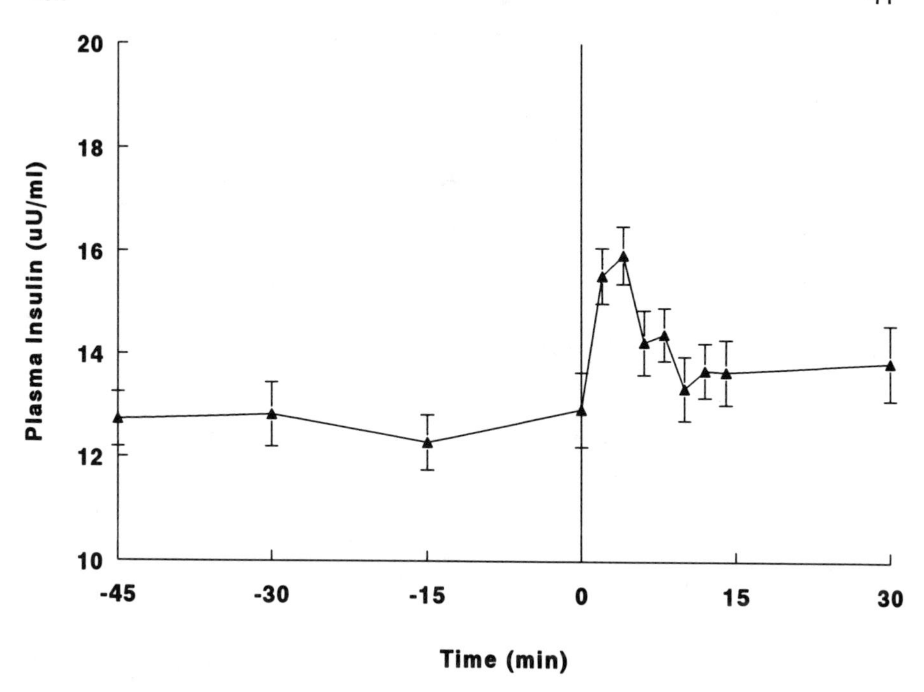


**FIGURE 1.** Mean ± SE cephalic phase insulin release of 15 normal weight male subjects after a modified sham-feed. Subjects tasted, chewed, but did not swallow a peanut butter sandwich for a 2-min period. Sampling began immediately after the modified sham-feed.

onstrated CPIR with the nonnutritive sweetener saccharin[3,25] and also when nutritive sweeteners such as glucose or sucrose are administered to animals with gastric fistulas.[26,27] Due to the rapid absorption of simple sugars, nutritive sweeteners in significant amounts cannot be used as a stimulus without the possibility of direct glucose-stimulated insulin release. Therefore, in humans, one is usually limited to using nonnutritive sweeteners to explore the role of sweet taste as a stimulus for CPIR.

Only two studies have directly examined the effect of nonnutritive sweeteners on CPIR, each using a different sweetener and each reporting discrepant results. Porte et al.[8] orally administered a saccharin-sweetened solution and compared the effects on plasma insulin to either a control solution or saccharin administered intravenously. Significant increases in plasma insulin at 20 min postingestion were found after the orally administered saccharin. No significant increases were observed during the other two conditions. In contrast, Bruce et al.[13] found no significant increase in plasma insulin when subjects drank an aspartame-flavored solution. Preliminary results from our laboratory (Figure 3) suggest that a cherry-flavored beverage sweetened with aspartame does not elicit CPIR. However,

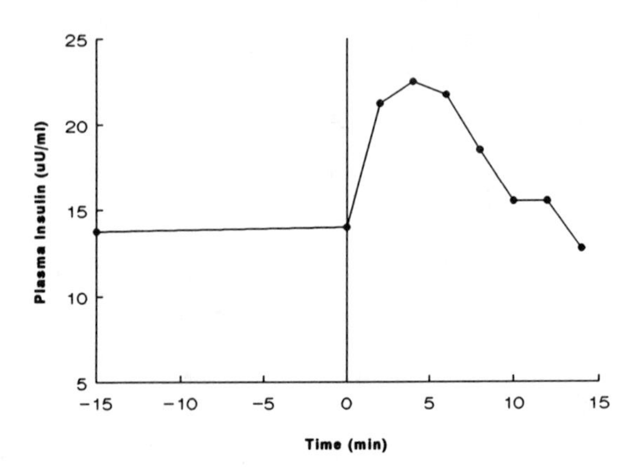


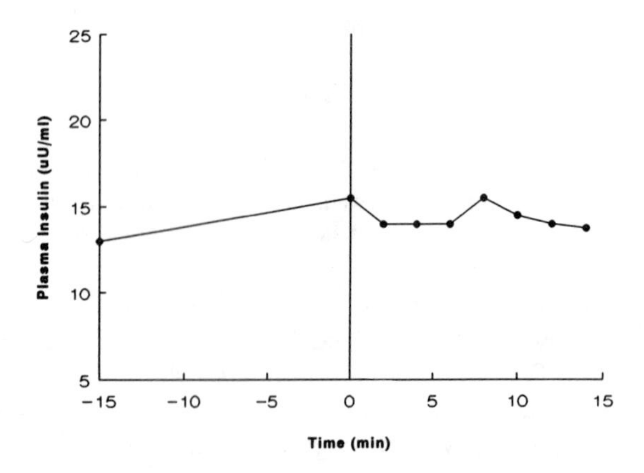


**FIGURE 2.** Upper graph represents a typical profile of cephalic phase insulin release in an individual subject. Lower graph represents a lack of response in an individual considered to be a "nonresponder".

when subjects consume the beverage with a peanut butter sandwich, CPIR is observed. It is difficult to reconcile why a palatable, sweet solution is not a sufficient stimulus to elicit CPIR. Perhaps beverages are not usually coupled with caloric consumption and, therefore, due to either conditioning or cognitive associations, CPIR does not occur. Alternatively, textural stimulation combined with chewing may be required to elicit the response in humans. Obviously, more detailed experiments are required to determine the effectiveness of sweet taste as a stimulus for CPIR and to examine if

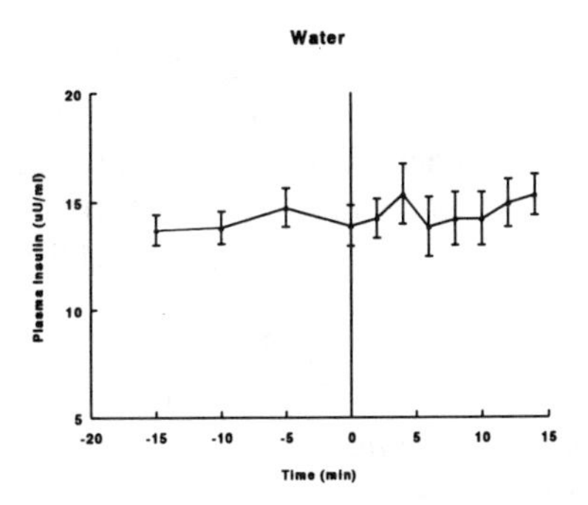


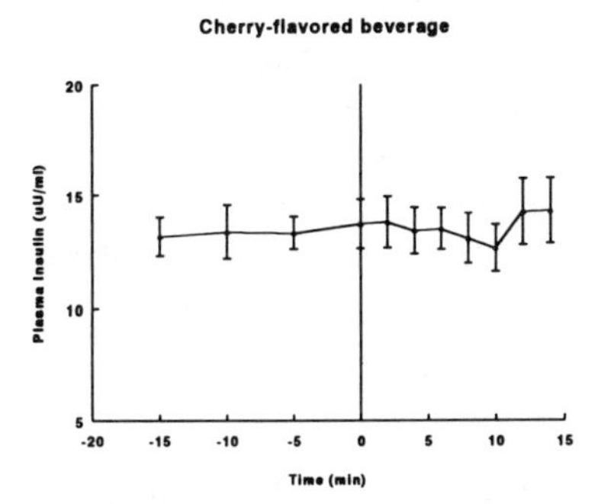


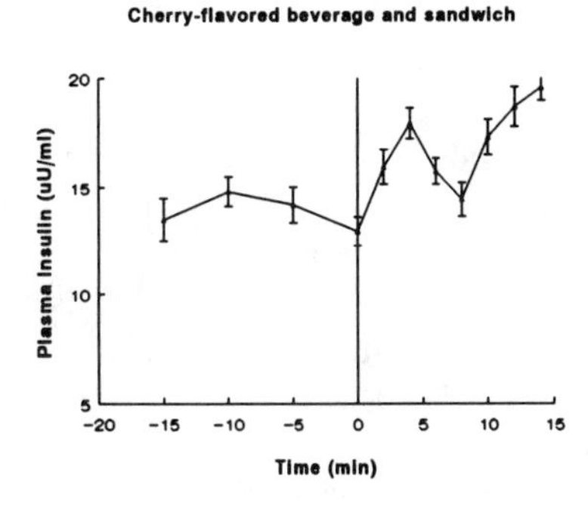


**FIGURE 3.** Mean ± SE cephalic phase insulin release of 10 normal weight men after consumption of (1) water (upper graph), (2) cherry-flavored beverage sweetened with aspartame (middle graph), and (3) cherry-flavored beverage sweetened with aspartame and a peanut butter sandwich.

there are differences in the effectiveness of nonnutritive sweeteners to elicit CPIR in humans.

In general, the optimal sensory stimuli required to elicit CPIR have not been established. A review of the existing literature suggests that there is a correlation between the complexity of the sensory stimulus and its efficacy in stimulating CPIR. Therefore, food ingestion that involves visual, olfactory, and gustatory stimuli is more effective than visual and olfactory stimulation by itself. However, there is no information concerning the relationship between diet composition or quantity and the magnitude of CPIR. This will be an important area of future research, particularly once the physiological significance of CPIR is established.

### C. Physiological Significance of CPIR

Interest in the ability of a nonnutritive sweetener to stimulate the release of cephalic phase insulin was stimulated by the finding that consumption of aspartame-sweetened solutions was associated with an increased sensation of hunger in normal volunteers.[28,29] CPIR was suggested as a potential mechanism by which a sweet-tasting beverage could elicit hunger,[30,31] although, as discussed above, there is little evidence that a nonnutritive sweetener is capable of eliciting CPIR in humans. The idea of CPIR as an initiator of food intake was first put forward by Powley[2] in his "cephalic phase hypothesis", which suggested that heightened cephalic phase responses were responsible for the hyperphagia and, ultimately, the obesity observed in rats with lesions in the ventromedial hypothalamus (VMH). Louis-Sylvestre[32] subsequently demonstrated that obese rats did exhibit exaggerated CPIR as compared to normal weight animals while Berthoud et al.[3] reported that animals with relatively "high" CPIR gained more weight on a cafeteria diet than those animals with "low CPIR". Furthermore, rats with transplanted pancreatic islet cells that are not neurally innervated and do not exhibit CPIR eat smaller meals than control animals.[33] Additional support was provided by evidence that obese human subjects exhibited CPIR of greater magnitude than normal weight subjects.[18,19] However, some investigators[23,34] have argued that the increased magnitude of CPIR in obese animals and humans is solely a reflection of basal hyperinsulinemia, while others have demonstrated that the hyperphagia associated with VMH lesioned rats is not due to vagally mediated insulin release.[35]

In the cephalic phase hypothesis, it was also assumed that there existed a direct relationship between the magnitude of the cephalic phase reflexes and the palatability of the food stimulus, a relationship first reported by Pavlov.[1] In fact, with respect to CPIR, there is no conclusive evidence in humans that supports the animal data. Only two studies have attempted to address this question.[14,36] Both studies rendered food unpalatable by blending a combination of foods together and permitting subjects to ingest the blended food. Unpublished data from this laboratory have indicated that the rate of absorption of blended food is significantly faster than the consumption of the food in its entirety. Therefore, due to the rapid time frame of CPIR, comparisons between these two treatments are not possible. Thus, close examination of the literature reveals that the hypothesis suggesting that CPIR is an initiator of food intake is based on rather limited information. However, if the response is not regulating food intake, then what other physiological role could it play?

Traditionally, the cephalic phase reflexes are assumed to optimize the digestion and absorption of incoming nutrients. Various hypotheses have been put forward suggesting that the cephalic phase reflexes are adaptive responses designed to minimize the impact of nutrient influxes during a meal.[25,37,38] Woods[37] postulated that increased food consumption conditions learned increases in CPIR, thereby permitting physiological adjustment to greater nutrient loads. Thus, CPIR would act as a buffer to prevent large postprandial fluctuations in plasma insulin and glucose levels.[25,37] However, although this hypothesis is consistent with the general concept of cephalic phase reflexes, it is still not known if the magnitude of the response can be altered by dietary intake or even if the absolute magnitude is of physiological significance. If one considers the total amount of insulin released during the cephalic phase time period, it does not appear to be of sufficient quantity to significantly alter plasma glucose levels. Alternatively, it may be that the absolute magnitude of the response is not important but that any increase in insulin during the very early period after ingestion is a sufficient stimulus or signal to initiate subsequent mechanisms responsible for optimal glucose metabolism.

The physiological effects of an absence or inhibition of CPIR reflect the importance of the response despite its relatively small magnitude. Both animal and human work demonstrate that manipulations that prevent or inhibit CPIR result in hyperglycemia and subsequent hyperinsulinemia.[39-42] In animals, bypassing the oropharyngeal receptors by intragastric administration of glucose results in decreased glucose tolerance when compared to oral ingestion.[39] Similarly in humans, inhibition of early insulin release by the administration of somatostatin to normal volunteers from –5 to 15 min during an oral glucose tolerance test also results in a deterioration of glucose tolerance and an increased insulin release in contrast to a saline control.[40] Therefore, the absence of CPIR results in abnormal glucose metabolism. Storlein and Bruce[38] suggested that impaired CPIR due to learned or genetic abnormalities could lead to postprandial hyperglycemia and hyperinsulinemia, particularly in the obese, thereby contributing to the development of diabetes mellitus. This hypothesis is consistent with the effects of inhibition of CPIR, but to date, there has been no evidence of impaired CPIR in humans. We have recently completed a study comparing CPIR in normal weight and obese subjects.[23] In contrast to previously published reports (Table 2), we found a trend toward attenuated CPIR in the obese as compared to normal weight subjects when the data were expressed as a percentage of basal insulin levels. Moreover, due to the elevated levels of fasting insulin in many of the obese subjects, we felt it was important to establish that increases in CPIR were independent of a basal hypersecretion of insulin. We then divided the obese population into two groups: (1) subjects with normal levels of fasting insulin and (2) subjects with elevated levels of fasting insulin. By this method, we demonstrated that both groups of obese subjects exhibited a trend toward attenuated CPIR when expressed as a percent of basal insulin. However, when the data were expressed as an absolute difference from baseline, the method commonly used in other studies, only the hyperinsulinemic group exhibited exaggerated CPIR. These findings supported the argument that the increased magnitude of CPIR reported in the obese is merely a reflection of basal hyperinsulinemia. Interestingly, obese subjects with normal levels of fasting insulin still exhibited the attenuation in CPIR and also expressed a hyperinsulinemic postprandial response. Whether the impaired CPIR contributes to the postprandial hyperinsulinemia observed in the obese subjects is not known. However, as discussed above, it seems unlikely that the absolute magnitude of CPIR could account for the abnormality in glucose metabolism. Therefore, one must consider the potential mechanisms by which CPIR could alter glucose homeostasis.

One hypothesis suggests that CPIR may be acting directly on hepatic glucose metabolism by inhibiting gluconeogenesis or by altering the activity of hepatic enzymes that are involved in regulating plasma glucose levels.[38] As the concentration of insulin in the hepatic portal vein is twice that found in the peripheral circulation, the liver is receiving a sharp, rapid increase of insulin that is of greater magnitude than in other tissues. Therefore, the liver is a likely recipient of the CPIR signal. An alternate possibility is that CPIR stimulates afferent receptors in the liver,[43] thereby relaying information to the central nervous system (CNS) that ultimately alters peripheral metabolism. The role of the CNS in glucoregulation has been well documented.[44,45] Electrical stimulation of specific brain areas such as the nucleus of the solitary tract and the ventromedial hypothalamus has been shown to alter hepatic glucose metabolism as well as pancreatic insulin secretion. Administration of atropine inhibits the effects on both tissues and emphasizes the importance of vagal stimulation.[44,45] In fact, cholinergic activation appears to be crucial in both hepatic glucose metabolism and in the optimization of insulin secretion from the pancreas. For example, *in vitro* studies have shown that islet cells preexposed to cholinergic agonists release more insulin than nonexposed islets.[46] Furthermore, stimulation of the vagus nerve increases glycogen synthetase activity and, hence, deposition of liver glycogen.[47] Therefore, vagal activity that can be elicited through oral sensory stimulation initiates a series of physiological responses that may be of individual physiological significance or may be acting in concert as preparatory reflexes. When oral sensory stimulation does not take place, for example, after intragastric or intravenous administration of glucose, vagal activation does not occur and results in submaximal glucose metabolism and an exaggerated release of post-prandial insulin.[48,49]

## III. SUMMARY

The importance of oral sensory stimulation in the optimization of nutrient absorption and digestion has been well documented since the turn of the century. The early release of the anabolic hormone insulin that occurs during sensory stimulation and is termed cephalic phase insulin release may play a role in the regulation of glucose homeostasis as impairment of the response results in hyperglycemia and subsequent hyperinsulinemia. However, in humans, there still remain many unanswered questions concerning the sensory stimuli required to elicit the response and the mechanisms by which the release of such a small quantity of insulin could influence blood glucose levels.

## REFERENCES

1. Pavlov, I., *The Work of the Digestive Glands,* Charles Griffin, London, 1902.
2. Powley, T. L., The ventromedial hypothalamic syndrome, satiety and a cephalic phase hypothesis, *Psychol. Rev.,* 84, 89, 1977.
3. Berthoud, H. R., Bereiter, D. A., Trimble, E. R., Siegel, E. G., and Jeanrenaud, B., Cephalic phase, reflex insulin secretion, *Diabetologia,* 20, 393, 1981.
4. Feldman, M., and Richardson, C. T., Role of thought, sight, smell and taste of food in the cephalic phase of gastric acid secretion in humans, *Gastroenterology,* 90, 428, 1986.
5. Janowitz, H. D., Hollander, F., Orringer, D., Levy, M. H., Winkelstein, A., Kaufman, R., and Margolim, S. G., A quantitative study of the gastric secretory response to sham-feeding in a human subject, *Gastroenterology,* 16, 104, 1950.
6. Richardson, C. T., and Feldman, M., Salivary response to food in humans and its effect on gastric acid secretion, *Am. J. Physiol.,* 250, G85, 1986.
7. Goldfine, I. D., Abraira, C., Gruenwald, D., and Goldstein, M. S., Plasma insulin levels during imaginary food ingestion under hypnosis, *Proc. Soc. Exp. Biol. Med.,* 133, 274, 1970.
8. Porte, D., Jr., Robertson, R. P., Halter, J. B., Kulkosky, P. J., Makous, W. L., and Woods, S. C., Neuroendocrine recognition of glucose: the glucoreceptor hypothesis and the diabetic syndrome. In: *Food Intake and Chemical Senses,* Y. Katsubi, M. Sato, S. F. Tabogi, and Y. Oomura, Eds. University Park Press, Baltimore, 1977, 336.
9. Sahakian, B. J., Lean, M. E. J., Robbins, T. W., and James, W. P. T., Salivation and insulin secretion in response to food in non-obese men and women, *Appetite,* 2, 209, 1981.

10. Bellisle, F., Louis-Sylvestre, J., Demozay, F., Blazy, D., and Le Magnen, J., Reflex insulin response associated to food intake in human subjects, *Physiol. Behav.,* 31, 515, 1983.
11. Bellisle, F., Louis-Sylvestre, J., Demozay, F., Blazy, D., and Le Magnen, J., Cephalic phase of insulin secretion and food stimulation in humans, *Am. J. Physiol.,* 249, E638, 1985.
12. Yamazaki, M., and Sakaguchi, T., Effects of d-glucose anomers on sweetness taste and insulin release in man, *Brain Res. Bull.,* 17, 271, 1986.
13. Bruce, D. G., Storlein, L. H., Furler, S. M., and Chisholm, D. J., Cephalic phase metabolic responses in normal weight adults, *Metabolism,* 36, 721, 1987.
14. Lucas, F., Bellisle, F., and Di Maio, A., Spontaneous insulin fluctuations and the preabsorptive insulin response to food ingestion in humans, *Physiol. Behav.,* 40, 631, 1987.
15. Teff, K. L., Mattes, R. D., and Engelman, K., Cephalic phase insulin release in normal weight males: verification and reliability, *Am. J. Physiol.,* 261, E430, 1991.
16. Teff, K. L., Levin, B., and Engelman, K., Oral sensory stimulation in men: effects on insulin, c-pepticle and colecholamines. *Am. J. Physiol.,* In press.
17. Parra-Covarubias, A., Rivera-Rodriguez, I., and Almaraz-Ugalde, A., Cephalic phase of insulin secretion in obese adolescents, *Diabetes,* 20, 800, 1972.
18. Rodin, J., Has the distinction between internal versus external control of feeding behavior outlived its usefulness? In: *Recent Advances in Obesity Research,* G. A. Bray, Ed. Neuman Press, London, 1978, 79.
19. Sjostrom, L., Garelick, G., Krotkiewski, M., and Luyckx, A., Peripheral insulin in response to the sight and smell of food, *Metabolism,* 29, 901, 1980.
20. Johnson, W. G., and Wildman, H. E., Influence of external and covert food stimuli on insulin secretion in obese and normal persons, *Behav. Neurosci.,* 97, 1025, 1983.
21. Osuna, J. I., Pages, I., Motino, M. A., Rodriguez, E., and Osorio, C., Cephalic phase of insulin secretion in obese women, *Horm. Metabol. Res.,* 18, 473, 1986.
22. Simon, C., Schlienger, J. L., Sapin, R., and Imler, M., Cephalic phase insulin secretion in relation to food presentation in normal and overweight subjects, *Physiol. Behav.,* 36, 465, 1986.
23. Teff, K. L., Mattes, R. D., Engelman, K. and Mattern, J. Cephalic phase insulin release in obese and normal weight men: relation to postprondial insulin. *Metabolism,* In press.
24. Taylor, I. L., and Feldman, M., Effect of cephalic-vagal stimulation on insulin, gastric inhibitory polypeptide, and pancreatic polypeptide release in humans, *J. Clin. Endocrin. Metabol.,* 55, 1114, 1982.
25. Nicolaidis, S., Early systemic responses to oro-gastric stimulation in the regulation of food and water imbalance. Functional and electrophysiological data, *Ann. N.Y. Acad. Sci.,* 157, 1176, 1969.
26. Strubbe, J. H., and Steffens, A. B., Rapid insulin release after ingestion of a meal in the unanaesthetized rat, *Am. J. Physiol.,* 229, 1019, 1975.

27. Grill, H. J., Berridge, K., and Ganster, D. J., Oral glucose is the prime elicitor of preabsorptive insulin secretion, *Am. J. Physiol.,* 246, R88, 1984.
28. Blundell, J. E., and Hill, A., J. Paradoxical effects of an intense sweetener (aspartame) on appetite, *Lancet,* 1, 1092, 1986.
29. Rogers, P. J., Carlyle, J., Hill, A. J., and Blundell, J. E., Uncoupling sweet taste and calories: comparison of the effects of glucose and three intense sweeteners on hunger and food intake, *Physiol. Behav.,* 43, 547, 1988.
30. Rogers, P. J., and Blundell, J. E., Separating the actions of sweeteness and calories: effects of saccharin and carbohydrates on hunger and food intake in human subjects, *Physiol. Behav.,* 45, 1093, 1989.
31. Black, R. M., Tanaka, P., Leiter, L., and Anderson, G. H., Soft drinks with aspartame: effect on subjective hunger, food selection, and food intake of young adult males, *Physiol. Behav.,* 49, 803, 1991.
32. Louis-Sylvestre, J., Preabsorptive insulin release and hypoglycemia in rats, *Am. J. Physiol.,* 230, 56, 1976.
33. Inoue, S., Bray, G., and Mullen, Y. S., Transplantation of pancreatic B-cells prevents development of hypothalamic obesity in rats, *Am. J. Physiol.,* 235, E277, 1978.
34. Storlein, L. H., The role of the ventromedial hypothalamic area in periprandial glucoregulation, *Life Sci.,* 36, 505, 1985.
35. Scalfani, A., The role of hyperinsulinemia and the vagus nerve in hypothalamic hyperphagia reexamined, *Diabetologia,* 20, 402, 1981.
36. Leblanc, J., and Brondel, L., Role of palatability on meal-induced thermogenesis in human subjects, *Am. J. Physiol.,* 248, E333, 1985.
37. Woods, S. C., The eating paradox: how we tolerate food, *Psychol. Rev.,* 98, 488, 1991.
38. Storlein, L. H., and Bruce, D. G., Mind over metabolism: the cephalic phase in relation to non-insulin dependent diabetes and obesity, *Biol. Psych.,* 28, 3, 1989.
39. Proietto, J., Rohner-Jeanrenaud, F., Ionescu, E., and Jeanrenaud, B., Role of the oropharynx in regulation of glycemia, *Diabetes,* 36, 791, 1987.
40. Calles-Escandon, J., and Robbins, D. C., Loss of early phase of insulin release in humans impairs glucose intolerance and blunts thermic effect of glucose, *Diabetes,* 36, 1167, 1987.
41. Bruce, D. G., Chisholm, D. J., Storlein, L. H., and Kraegen, E. W., Physiological importance of deficiency in early prandial insulin secretion in non-insulin dependent diabetes, *Diabetes,* 37, 736, 1988.
42. Kraegen, E. W., Chisholm, D. J., and McNamara, M. E., Timing of insulin delivery with meals, *Horm. Metab. Res.,* 13, 365, 1981.
43. Niijima, A., Glucose-sensitive afferent nerve fibres in the hepatic branch of the vagus nerve in the guinea-pig, *J. Physiol.,* 33, 315, 1982.
44. Shimazu, T., Central nervous system regulation of liver and adipose tissue metabolism, *Diabetologia,* 20, 343, 1981.
45. Steffens, A. B., Strubbe, J. H., Balkan, B., and Scheurink, A. J. W., Neuroendocrine mechanisms involved in regulation of body weight, food intake and metabolism, *Neurosci. Biobehav. Rev.,* 14, 305, 1990.

46. Zawalich, W. S., Zawalich, K. C., and Rasmussen, H., Cholinergic agonists prime the B-cell to glucose stimulation, *Endocrinology,* 125, 2400, 1989.
47. Shimazu, T., Regulation of glycogen metabolism in liver by the autonomic nervous system. V. Activation of glycogen synthetase by vagal stimulation, *Biochim. Biophys. Acta.,* 252, 28, 1971.
48. Erlick, H., Stimmler, L., Hlad, C. J., and Arai, Y., Plasma insulin response to oral and intravenous glucose administration, *J. Clin. Endocrinol.,* 24, 1076, 1964.
49. Hampton, S. M., Morgan, L. M., Tredger, J. A., Cramb, R., and Marks, V., Insulin and C-peptide levels after oral and intravenous glucose, *Diabetes,* 35, 612, 1986.

# 4 The Effect of Dietary Macronutrients on Brain Serotonin Formation

John D. Fernstrom

## I. INTRODUCTION

The brain receives numerous forms of sensory information during food ingestion, digestion, and absorption, including data on smell, taste, texture, and composition. Such information appears to be important in determining what and when the animal will eat, and how the body will handle food metabolically. It is not difficult to appreciate intuitively how and why smell, taste, and texture impact on food selection and intake. It is more difficult, however, to understand the manner in which food composition (particularly the macronutrient composition) impacts on food choice. Such effects are presumed to be elaborated, at least in part, at the metabolic level. Over the years, various hypotheses have been examined to identify metabolic signals that inform the brain about recent food acquisition. One such hypothesis considers circulating amino acids to be important signals. Work in our laboratory has focused on a particular group of amino acids, the large neutral amino acids (LNAA), for two reasons: first, two of the LNAA (tryptophan [TRP] and tyrosine [TYR]) are precursors of brain neurotransmitters (serotonin [5HT] and the catecholamines, respectively), and alterations in their uptake into brain have been shown to influence directly their rates of conversion to neurotransmitter products.[1] And second, because *all* of the circulating LNAA compete for uptake into brain via a shared transport carrier located at the blood-brain barrier, variations in the blood level of any LNAA can ultimately influence the production of 5HT and the catecholamines. When changes in precursor level influence transmitter synthesis, they also influence transmitter release from neurons,[2] which could well influence the activity of brain circuits involved in the control of food intake.

0-8493-4466-2/94/$0.00+$.50

Two macronutrients, carbohydrate and protein, are known to influence 5HT and catecholamine production via this mechanism. Some data suggest fat intake might also be expected to influence TRP uptake into brain and 5HT production, though the mechanism does not involve competitive LNAA transport into brain.[3] This chapter will focus on the relationship of TRP supply to 5HT synthesis. Information regarding the relationship of CNS TYR uptake and catecholamine synthesis has recently been reviewed elsewhere.[1]

## II. TRYPTOPHAN SUPPLY AND SEROTONIN SYNTHESIS IN BRAIN

Serotonin is synthesized from TRP, an essential amino acid, in a two-step reaction. TRP is first hydroxylated to 5-hydroxytryptophan (5HTP), a reaction catalyzed by TRP hydroxylase. 5HTP is then decarboxylated to 5HT in a reaction mediated by aromatic-L-amino acid decarboxylase. The hydroxylation step is rate-limiting, suggesting that controls on the pathway will be focused on TRP hydroxylation (Figure 1).[4] The activity of TRP hydroxylase is undoubtedly governed by multiple control mechanisms. However, one mechanism that is of particular interest physiologically is the level of substrate. TRP hydroxylase is normally not fully saturated with TRP; indeed, normal brain TRP levels approximate the $K_m$ for this enzyme. As a result, the rate of TRP hydroxylation (and thus 5HT synthesis) varies rapidly and directly with changes in brain TRP levels,[5,6] particularly when 5HT neurons are active.[2,7]

TRP levels in brain, in turn, appear to be rapidly responsive to changes in TRP uptake from the circulation, which is mediated by a competitive transport carrier TRP shares with several other LNAA (e.g., TYR, phenylalanine, leucine, isoleucine, valine).[8] As a consequence, brain TRP uptake (and thus brain TRP levels and 5HT synthesis) can be influenced by changes in the blood levels of TRP or any of the other LNAA.[9] For example, brain TRP levels can rise either when blood TRP increases or the levels of its competitors fall. Conversely, brain TRP falls when blood TRP declines, or the blood levels of the other LNAA rise. The earliest application of these observations was in a dietary context: if a fasting rat consumed a carbohydrate meal, blood TRP levels were observed to rise, while the levels of the other LNAA fell (the result of insulin secretion and action). These changes favored a rise in brain TRP uptake; indeed, brain TRP levels were increased (and 5HT synthesis was stimulated[10]). If the rat consumed a meal containing protein in addition to carbohydrate, blood TRP again rose significantly, but instead of the other LNAA falling, their blood levels also rose, if the dietary protein content was high (in this case, the dietary LNAA more than offset the insulin-induced drop in blood LNAA levels). In fact, the blood levels of

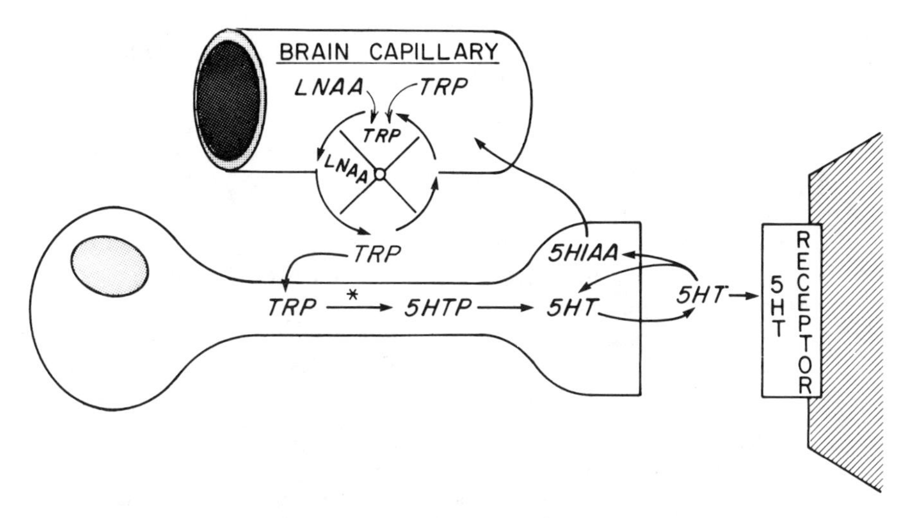


**FIGURE 1.** Tryptophan (TRP) availability and serotonin (5HT) synthesis. Tryptophan is converted to 5HT by a two-step, enzymatic reaction (see text). Monoamine oxidase initiates the catabolism of 5HT to 5-hydroxyindoleacetic acid (5HIAA). Asterisk indicates rate-limiting step in 5HT formation, TRP hydroxylation. TRP competes with other large, neutral amino acids (LNAA) for uptake into brain.

TRP and its competitors were observed to rise by proportionally similar amounts. As a result, brain TRP uptake and levels, and 5HT synthesis were unchanged.[10] For convenience, the changes in the plasma LNAA pattern produced by such meals that are relevant to brain TRP uptake can be expressed as a ratio of the serum TRP concentration divided by the sum of the concentrations of the other LNAA (TRP/ΣLNAA). Thus, carbohydrate ingestion raises this ratio, while the consumption of carbohydrates with a significant level of dietary protein does not.[10]

## III. PROTEIN AND CARBOHYDRATE INGESTION AND BRAIN SEROTONIN SYNTHESIS

Over the past 20 years, many interesting implications and extensions of this set of relationships have been examined in a variety of physiological and pathophysiological states. The physiological implication most frequently advanced has been that meal-induced changes in brain TRP levels and 5HT production inform the brain about the most recent meal's carbohydrate and/or protein contents. As a consequence, this set of relationships is said to be important in the regulation of carbohydrate and/or protein intake from meal to meal.[11-14] While this is an appealing concept, it depends on brain TRP uptake and 5HT production changing with the ingestion of each meal. Is this a reasonable expectation? The original studies fed rats a single meal following an overnight fast,[10] a design that would insure a robust increase in blood insulin levels over a low, fasting value. Perhaps these changes would be blunted in a second or third meal, separated by only a few hours (as would normally be the case in humans). As a result, the meal-induced effects would disappear with succeeding meals, seriously compromising any such models of food intake regulation.

Recent data obtained in our laboratory suggest that meal-induced changes in brain TRP uptake and 5HT synthesis *can* continue to respond to the repetitive ingestion of food. We have examined brain TRP levels and 5HT synthesis in rats that have ingested two meals separated by 2 h. For example, when rats were fasted overnight, and presented with a small meal of carbohydrates (the meal size was about 20% of the rat's daily caloric intake), brain TRP levels and 5HT synthesis rose 2 h later (Figure 2), as expected. If animals fed this initial carbohydrate meal received a second meal of the same caloric size at 2 h, containing 40% protein, brain TRP levels and 5HT synthesis returned to fasting values by the time they were killed (2 h later). If the second meal was carbohydrates alone, brain TRP and 5HT remained elevated (Figure 2). In other studies, in which protein meals were presented first, followed by carbohydrate meals, the second meal would raise brain TRP and 5HT within 2 h, but only if the protein content of the first meal was not too great (less than about 12% protein). Apparently, plasma LNAA levels following a large protein meal remain high enough long enough that the insulin secreted in response to a carbohydrate meal 2 h later cannot lower their levels sufficiently to allow brain TRP to rise.

From these results, it is apparent that brain TRP uptake and 5HT synthesis can indeed continue to respond to repeated meals, *but within metabolic limits that make some sense*. For example, when the first meal is carbohydrates alone, and brain TRP and 5HT rise, a second meal of moderate to high protein content will probably reduce brain TRP and 5HT, even if consumed soon after the first meal: the introduction of the new LNAA from the meal should raise blood levels of the LNAA sufficiently to lower brain TRP (Figure 2). However, if the second meal contains small amounts of protein, its ingestion soon after the first meal may not raise blood LNAA levels, and thus brain TRP uptake may not fall. The same meal, though, ingested after a longer intermeal interval, might then be able to raise blood LNAA levels sufficiently to reduce brain TRP (because insulin effects would have diminished). Conversely, if a large protein meal were the first meal to be consumed, and as a result brain TRP and 5HT remained low, the timing of a second, carbohydrate meal would be quite important in determining its ability to raise brain TRP and 5HT: insulin secretion would be the only

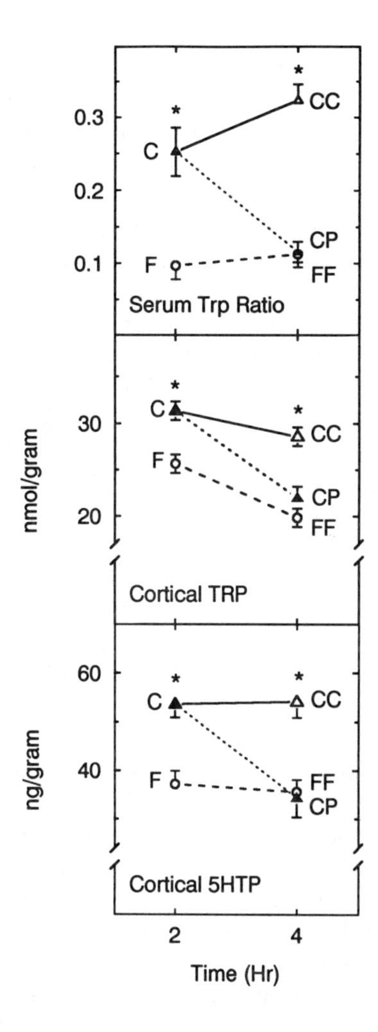


**FIGURE 2.** Effect of the ingestion of two sequential meals on brain tryptophan levels and 5HT synthesis. Groups of seven male rats, fasted overnight, ingested at 0 h (0900) either nothing, or 8 g of a carbohydrate diet (C). Ninety minutes later, one group of fasting rats and one group fed carbohydrate received an i.p. injection of *m*-hydroxybenzylhydrazine (NSD-1015, an inhibitor of aromatic-L-amino acid decarboxylase), and were killed 30 min later at 2 h. At 2 h, other groups of rats fed an initial carbohydrate meal received a second meal, consisting of either 8 g of carbohydrates or 8 g of a 40% protein diet; a group of fasting rats continued to fast. Ninety minutes after the second meal was presented, all remaining rats received NSD-1015, and were killed 30 min thereafter at 4 h. The data are presented at the means ± SEM. *$p$ <0.01 vs. fasting values at the same time point (2 h, $t$ test; 4 h, Newman-Keuls test). F, FF = fasting; C = one carbohydrate meal; CP = carbohydrate meal followed by a 40% protein meal; CC = two sequential carbohydrate meals (M. H. Fernstrom, and J. D. Fernstrom, unpublished observations).

response to the second meal causing blood LNAA levels to change. The longer the intermeal interval, the more likely a rise in brain TRP uptake would result from the ingestion of the second meal. As a corollary, a reduction in the necessary intermeal interval could be predicted as the protein content of the first meal was reduced.

If one were extrapolating to humans (for which the model was developed, since rats do not typically eat a few, large meals each day separated by several hours), some fairly straightforward predictions could be made. First, breakfast should be a meal at which the clearest effects on brain TRP and 5HT should be apparent (because of the overnight fast). If breakfast and lunch were separated by 3 to 4 h, then in the absence of morning snacks, lunch would probably also produce significant changes in brain TRP and 5HT (e.g., if breakfast was high carbohydrate, and lunch high protein, lunch might reduce brain TRP uptake and 5HT production). A breakfast of modest size would further promote metabolic responsivity at lunch. However, if the breakfast were large, of high-protein content, and separated from lunch by only a few hours, then the blood LNAA responses to lunch might not be remarkable. A similar set of arguments can be made for the separation of lunch and dinner; an afternoon snack might become important, depending on its caloric size and protein content.

Given this level of complexity, one might ask if this set of nutritional, metabolic, and neurochemical relationships could serve as a useful signal to brain regarding recent ingestion of protein or carbohydrate. Certainly, with meals separated by at least a few hours, the repeated ingestion of high-protein meals should keep brain 5HT lower than after the ingestion of multiple carbohydrate-rich/very-low-protein meals. The repeated ingestion of meals containing intermediate levels of protein might center brain TRP uptake between these two dietary opposites. Such is certainly suggested indirectly by the results of dietary studies in humans.[15] Moreover, a meal of carbohydrates consumed by individuals ingesting on average large amounts of protein in their meals (e.g., 100–150 g/day) might produce a clear spike in brain 5HT against a background of lower brain 5HT levels, and thus clearly indicate to the brain that a high carbohydrate meal had been ingested. The converse should also be true. Thus, the answer to the question may indeed be yes, both in the context of chronic diet and single meals. However, such evidence *alone* does *not* constitute proof that the brain actually senses protein or carbohydrate ingestion (or both) by this mechanism.

How might these considerations influence thoughts about appetite regulation, particularly as relates to protein and carbohydrate ingestion? The present data could probably be used to support most current notions regarding a role for brain 5HT neurons in the control of carbohydrate or protein intake. However, taking the notion of carbohydrate intake regulation as an example, the present results add only supportive, *not* definitive information.

The model must stand on more fundamental issues, such as (1) is there a metabolic requirement for carbohydrate in the diet; (2) is there any evidence that carbohydrate intake shows regulation over time (as evidenced by some degree of constancy of intake in the natural setting); and (3) is there evidence that carbohydrate intake is defended when it becomes scarce in the environment? The answer to each of these questions appears to be no for carbohydrate,[16] though data are by no means complete. A more positive argument can be made for protein,[13] though here too, information on intake appears to be thin. Until a detailed study is made of the natural patterns of intake of normal foods over an extended period of time, it will not be possible to make a convincing argument regarding the existence of systems for controlling the intake of any macronutrient, much less define the role of meal-induced changes in brain 5HT production and release within such control systems.

## IV. FAT INGESTION AND BRAIN SEROTONIN SYNTHESIS

The above studies focus on dietary protein and carbohydrates. Does the third macronutrient, fat, have any impact on brain TRP uptake and 5HT synthesis? Since fat ingestion is not a potent stimulus for insulin secretion, and does not appreciably influence circulating LNAA levels, one would not *a priori* predict major effects of fat intake on the competitive uptake of TRP into brain or on 5HT synthesis. However, there is a different mechanism by which dietary fat can be postulated to influence TRP access to the brain, involving the binding of TRP to albumin in blood. TRP is the only amino acid that circulates in blood bound to protein. About 70% of the blood TRP pool associates loosely with serum albumin; the remainder circulates as free TRP.[17] Because of this fact, several laboratories have argued that the free TRP fraction in blood is the biologically important TRP pool, and should dictate how much of the amino acid is accessible to brain transport carriers.[18,19] Thus, changes in the serum-free TRP pool should be rapidly reflected in parallel alterations in brain TRP uptake and levels, and thus in 5HT synthesis. Data offered in support of this notion include pharmacologic studies using agents that cause a substantial degree of unbinding of TRP from albumin,[20] as well as physiologic studies in which fasting, stress, or exercise was reported to cause TRP to disassociate from albumin, and lead to increments in brain TRP and 5HT.[3,21,22] The mechanism by which these treatments cause TRP to detach from albumin involves their ability to raise circulating levels of the nonesterified fatty acids (NEFA). NEFA compete with TRP for binding sites on the albumin molecule.[17] Thus, by raising blood NEFA levels, the above treatments cause TRP to be released from albumin binding sites, thereby raising serum-free TRP levels.

Serum NEFA levels can also be manipulated in rats by dietary means. Feeding rats a no-fat meal, for example, lowers serum NEFA levels;[23] feeding them a high-fat meal increases serum NEFA levels.[24] Thus, the relationship of circulating NEFA levels and free TRP levels to brain TRP and 5HT can be examined in rats using a nonstressful, nonpharmacologic procedure, food ingestion. Indeed, if the above studies are correct, brain 5HT synthesis should bear a direct relationship to a meal's fat content, and thus perhaps provide a clear signal to the brain regarding the amount of fat that has most recently been consumed. However, in early studies, when carbohydrate meals were fed to rats, they produced rapid reductions in serum NEFA and free TRP levels, but increases in brain TRP and 5HT.[23,25] Rats were also fed meals of varying fat contents, all containing high levels of protein.[24] Serum NEFA levels fell with the ingestion of low- or no-fat meals, but rose with the ingestion of high-fat meals. However, in no case was brain TRP altered vs. fasting, no doubt because of the inclusion of protein in all meals (which would raise blood levels of total TRP and the other LNAA, and swamp out any effects that might result from small changes in the free TRP pool).

While results such as these were interpreted as suggesting that dietary fat and free TRP levels were unimportant as determinants of brain TRP uptake, they did not actually resolve this issue. For example, the finding that variations in free TRP levels do not affect brain TRP when the blood levels of the LNAA are very high (because of protein ingestion) does not prove the notion that the free TRP changes are unimportant. It simply shows that under this particular condition the presence of high levels of competitors dominated the meal's impact on brain TRP uptake. Under dietary conditions in which blood LNAA levels do not vary, but free TRP does, the results might support the free TRP pool-brain TRP uptake hypothesis.

We have recently examined this issue using an experimental design that causes large changes in serum-free TRP levels following meal consumption, but no changes in the serum levels of the LNAA.[26] The model involves the use of diabetic (i.e., non-insulin-secreting) rats, and the feeding of nonprotein meals, since insulin secretion and dietary protein are the two dominant factors causing serum LNAA levels to change following food ingestion.[9] When fasting diabetic rats are fed a nonprotein, high-fat meal, serum-free TRP levels rise substantially, while serum total TRP levels and the levels of the other LNAA remain at pretreatment levels. A typical set of results of such studies is presented in Table 1. In this study, fasting diabetic rats consumed for 2 h a single meal containing either no fat (0% fat meal) or 45% fat (45% fat meal). The animals were all clearly diabetic, as indicated by the high fasting levels of serum glucose, and the very high glucose levels that followed the meal (five- to sixfold over normal values). Fasting serum concentrations of the LNAA were well within the normal

**TABLE 1**
**The Effects of Consuming a 0% Fat or 45% Fat Meal for 2 H on Serum and Brain Indices of TRP Uptake in Diabetic Rats[a]**

| | Fasting | 0% Fat meal | 45% Fat meal |
|---|---|---|---|
| Serum glucose (mg/100%) | 244 ± 38 | 708 ± 47* | 650 ± 65* |
| Serum NEFA (mEq/l) | 0.56 ± 0.10 | 0.75 ± 0.07 | 1.14 ± 0.11* |
| Serum total TRP (nmol/ml) | 120 ± 3 | 111 ± 5 | 111 ± 7 |
| Serum-free TRP (nmol/ml) | 23 ± 1 | 28 ± 1 | 56 ± 5* |
| Serum ΣLNAA (nmol/ml) | 754 ± 58 | 712 ± 66 | 726 ± 57 |
| Cortex TRP (nmol/g) | 19.5 ± 1.1 | 21.3 ± 0.2 | 20.9 ± 0.8 |
| Hypothalamus TRP (nmol/mg protein) | 0.248 ± 0.014 | 0.263 ± 0.009 | 0.255 ± 0.019 |

[a] Rats were fasted overnight and fed a diet for 2 h. Control rats continued to fast. Data represent the mean ± SEM ($n$ = 7/group).

* $p < 0.01$ vs. fasted controls (Newman–Keuls test).

Adapted from Fernstrom and Fernstrom.[26]

range. In response to the ingestion of the 45% fat meal, serum NEFA levels rose 2-fold, and serum free TRP levels about 2.5-fold. The levels of total TRP and the other LNAA (ΣLNAA), however, did not change from fasting values. Hence, this paradigm clearly set the animal up with a large, rapid increase in serum-free TRP levels, in the presence of *no* changes in the blood levels of its competitors for brain transport. The model should therefore produce a clear rise in brain TRP, if the free TRP pool is important in determining brain TRP uptake. However, TRP levels in two brain regions (hypothalamus and cerebral cortex) did not rise in those rats consuming the 45% fat meal, despite the large increments in serum-free TRP levels (Table 1). The same result was obtained if rats were studied 3 h after meal presentation.

At the very least, these results most clearly end any notion of a connection between meal-induced changes in serum-free TRP levels and alterations in brain TRP uptake (and thus 5HT synthesis). More generally, they also show there to be no link between dietary fat intake and brain 5HT synthesis. And, they again bring into question the whole notion that the circulating free TRP level is an important determinant of brain TRP uptake. Increases in serum free TRP were produced in these dietary studies that met and usually exceeded the magnitude of change in free TRP produced by other published procedures.[3,18,19,21] And yet, brain TRP levels did not change. One implication, therefore, is that the effects on brain TRP that occurred in these other studies followed from treatment effects other than those that occurred in the serum-free TRP pool. That is, the changes in serum-free TRP may have been *incidental* to the treatment-induced change in brain TRP uptake. Such a conclusion can certainly be drawn, for example, from the results of studies of another treatment that raised serum-free TRP and brain TRP levels, experimental hepatic cirrhosis.[27] The increase in brain TRP was shown to be related to increases in the activity of the TRP-LNAA transport carrier, not serum-free TRP.[28,29]

## V. CONCLUSIONS

The aim of this chapter has been to describe a particular biochemical–metabolic model by which food ingestion influences the synthesis of an important brain neurotransmitter, serotonin. The results show that meals of different carbohydrate and protein contents produce systematic, rapid alterations in brain TRP levels and 5HT synthesis. Such effects of single meals do not require that the animal be fasting for an extended period. Predictable changes in response to food ingestion occur when meals are separated by only a 2-h interval. The constituents of the meal that appear important in modifying brain TRP uptake and 5HT synthesis are protein and carbohydrate, acting by virtue of their effects on blood levels of TRP and other LNAA, and thus indirectly on the competitive transport of TRP into brain. The fat content of a meal appears unable to influence brain TRP levels or 5HT synthesis. When alterations in brain TRP levels produce parallel changes in 5HT synthesis, such as follows TRP administration, the release of 5HT from nerve terminals is similarly affected.[2] Meal-induced changes in brain TRP levels and 5HT synthesis thus probably modify 5HT release, thereby producing a biochemically identifiable effect on brain circuits containing 5HT neurons. Such changes in 5HT release may influence the overall activity of these circuits, some of which are thought to be involved in metabolic regulation and appetite control. However, while it is tempting to speculate further regarding the effects of such meal-induced changes in 5HT synthesis on brain circuits controlling appetite, it must be noted that no satisfactory model or data set presently exists that makes a convincing connection. Hopefully, with a more complete understanding of how meals influence TRP uptake and 5HT synthesis, better models will be forthcoming.

## VI. ACKNOWLEDGMENTS

The results described in this article were supported by a grant from the National Institutes of Health (HD-24730). The author is the recipient of an NIMH Research Scientist Award (MH-00254).

## REFERENCES

1. Fernstrom, J. D., Aromatic amino acids and monoamine synthesis in the central nervous system: Influence of the diet, *J. Nutr. Biochem.,* 1, 508, 1990.
2. Sharp, T., Bramwell, S. R., and Grahame-Smith, D. G., Effect of acute administration of L-tryptophan on the release of 5-HT in rat hippocampus in relation to serotoninergic neuronal activity: an in vivo microdialysis study, *Life Sci.,* 50, 1215, 1992.
3. Sarna, G. S., Katamaneni, B. D., and Curzon, G., Variables influencing the effect of a meal on brain tryptophan, *J. Neurochem.,* 44, 1575, 1985.
4. Cooper, J. R., Bloom, F. E., and Roth, R. H., *The Biochemical Basis of Neuropharmacology,* 6th Edition. Oxford University Press, New York, 1991.
5. Fernstrom, J. D., and Wurtman, R. J., Brain serotonin content: physiological dependence on plasma tryptophan levels, *Science,* 173, 149, 1971.
6. Ashcroft, G. W., Eccleston, D., and Crawford, T. B. B., 5-Hydroxyindole metabolism in rat brain. I. A study of intermediate metabolism using the technique of tryptophan loading, *J. Neurochem.,* 12, 483, 1965.
7. Fernstrom, M. H., Massoudi, M. S., and Fernstrom, J. D., Effect of 8-hydroxy-2-(di-n-propyl-amino)-tetralin on the tryptophan-induced increase in 5-hydroxytryptophan accumulation in rat brain, *Life Sci.,* 47, 283, 1990.
8. Pardridge, W. M., and Oldendorf, W. H., Kinetic analysis of blood brain barrier transport of amino acids, *Biochim. Biophys. Acta,* 401, 128, 1975.
9. Fernstrom, J. D., Role of precursor availability in the control of monoamine biosynthesis in brain, *Physiol. Rev.,* 63, 484, 1983.
10. Fernstrom, J. D., and Wurtman, R. J., Brain serotonin content: physiological regulation by plasma neutral amino acids, *Science,* 178, 414, 1972.
11. Wurtman, J. J., Neurotransmitter control of carbohydrate consumption, *Ann. N.Y. Acad. Sci.,* 443, 145, 1985.
12. Wurtman, R. J., Dietary treatments that affect brain neurotransmitters: effects on calorie and nutrient intake, *Ann. N.Y. Acad. Sci.,* 499, 179, 1987.
13. Anderson, G. H., Li, E. T. S., and Glanville, N. T., Brain mechanisms and the quantitative and qualitative aspects of food intake, *Brain Res. Bull.,* 12, 167, 1984.
14. Li, E. T. S., and Anderson, G. H., Self-selected meal composition, circadian rhythms and meal responses in plasma and brain tryptophan and 5-hydroxytryptamine in rats, *J. Nutr.,* 112, 2001, 1982.

15. Fernstrom, J. D., Wurtman, R. J., Hammarstrom Wiklund, B., Rand, W. M., Munro, H. N., and Davidson, C. S., Diurnal variations in plasma concentrations of tryptophan, tryosine, and other neutral amino acids: effect of dietary protein intake, *Am. J. Clin. Nutr.,* 32, 1912, 1979.
16. Fernstrom, J. D., Tryptophan, serotonin and carbohydrate appetite: will the real carbohydrate craver please stand up, *J. Nutr.,* 118, 1417, 1988.
17. McMenamy, R. H., and Oncley, J. L., The specific binding of L-tryptophan to serum albumin, *J. Biol. Chem.,* 233, 1436, 1958.
18. Tagliamonte, A., Biggio, G., Vargiu, L., and Gessa, G. L., Free tryptophan in serum controls brain tryptophan levels and serotonin synthesis, *Life Sci.,* 12(II), 277, 1973.
19. Knott, P. J., and Curzon, G., Free tryptophan in plasma and brain tryptophan metabolism, *Nature (London),* 239, 452, 1972.
20. Tagliamonte, A., Biggio, G., and Gessa, G. L., Possible role of "free" plasma tryptophan in controlling brain tryptophan concentrations, *Riv. Farmacol. Ter.,* 2, 251, 1971.
21. Chaouloff, F., Kennett, G. A., Serrurrier, B., Merino, D., and Curzon, G., Amino acid analysis demonstrates that increased plasma free tryptophan causes the increase of brain tryptophan during exercise in the rat, *J. Neurochem.,* 46, 1647, 1986.
22. Kennett, G. A., Curzon, G., Hunt, A., and Patel, A. J., Immobilization decreases amino acid concentrations in plasma but maintains or increases them in brain, *J. Neurochem.,* 46, 208, 1986.
23. Lipsett, D., Madras, B. K., Wurtman, R. J., and Munro, H. N., Serum tryptophan level after carbohydrate ingestion: selective decline in non-albumin-bound tryptophan coincident with reduction in serum free fatty acids, *Life Sci.,* 12(II), 57, 1973.
24. Madras, B. K., Cohen, E. L., Messing, R., Munro, H. N., and Wurtman, R. J., Relevance of free tryptophan in serum to tissue tryptophan concentrations, *Metabolism,* 23, 1107, 1974.
25. Madras, B. K., Cohen, E. L., Fernstrom, J. D., Larin, F., Munro, H. N., and Wurtman, R. J., Letter: Dietary carbohydrate increases brain tryptophan and decreases free plasma tryptophan, *Nature (London),* 244, 34, 1973.
26. Fernstrom, M. H., and Fernstrom, J. D., Large changes in serum free tryptophan levels do not alter brain tryptophan levels: studies in streptozotocin-diabetic rats, *Life Sci.,* 52, 907, 1993.
27. James, J. H., Hodgman, J. M., Funovics, J. M., Yoshimura, N., and Fischer, J. E., Brain tryptophan, plasma free tryptophan and distribution of plasma neutral amino acids, *Metabolism,* 25, 471, 1976.
28. James, J. H., Escourrou, J., and Fischer, J. E., Blood-brain neutral amino acid transport activity is increased after portacaval anastomosis, *Science,* 200, 1395, 1978.
29. Zanchin, G., Rigotti, P., Dussini, N., Vassanelli, P., and Battistin, L., Cerebral amino acid levels and uptake in rats after portocaval anastomosis. II. Regional studies in vivo, *J. Neurosci. Res.,* 4, 301, 1979.

# 5 Fuel Metabolism and Appetite Control

**Mark I. Friedman and Nancy E. Rawson**

The nervous system relies on a variety of sensory signals to control different aspects of feeding behavior.[1] Olfactory and gustatory stimuli are crucial for the recognition and selection of food, and stimuli from the gastrointestinal tract affect the size of a given meal. Signals associated with the postabsorptive processing of nutrients appear to be involved in meal initiation as well as the control of food consumption over longer intervals. These metabolic signals provide a link between energy homeostasis and short-term feeding behavior.

## I. AN INTEGRATED METABOLIC CONTROL OF FEEDING BEHAVIOR

For many years, food intake was thought to be controlled by separate signals generated in the metabolism of fat and glucose.[2] These "glucostatic" and "lipostatic" signals were believed to operate in a coordinated fashion, and this notion of a coordinated control has been used to account for a variety of fundamental phenomena, such as the relationship between body weight and feeding behavior, the diurnal rhythmicity of feeding, and maintenance of calorie intake.[2-4]

Evidence for a metabolic control of feeding behavior involving a mechanism that integrates information from fat and glucose metabolism comes in part from studies showing that different metabolic fuels are used interchangeably to control food intake. This use of alternative fuels is seen, for example, in the adjustment of food intake to compensate for caloric preloads or reductions in dietary calories independently of the source of calories (i.e., fat or carbohydrate).[5-7]

Direct evidence for an integrated metabolic control of feeding behavior stems from studies showing that combined reductions of fatty acid and glucose utilization produced by administration of metabolic inhibitors result in a greater eating response than would be expected from separate

0-8493-4466-2/94/$0.00+$.50

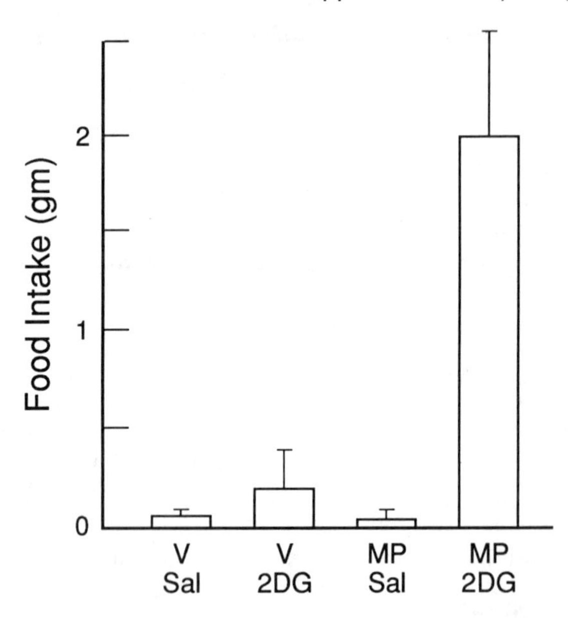


**FIGURE 1.** Synergistic increase in food intake of rats in response to combined inhibition of fatty acid oxidation and glucose utilization. Rats were given 10 mg/kg (p.o.) methyl palmoxirate (MP) to inhibit fatty acid oxidation or its vehicle (V), followed 2 h later by injection (i.p.) of either 100 mg/kg 2-deoxy-D-glucose (2DG) to inhibit glycolysis or saline (Sal).[8] Food intakes were measured 1 h after 2DG injection. Values are means ± SEM of 20 rats.

inhibition of the metabolism of each fuel.[8-13] In some cases, this interactive effect of combined blockade is observed even when metabolic inhibitors are given in doses that alone do not elicit eating (Figure 1).[8-10] Such a synergistic increase in food intake would not be observed if signals from glucose and fat metabolism controlled feeding independently, and indicate that changes in glucose and fat metabolism influence feeding via a common mechanism.

The nature of this integrative mechanism is an important question that must be answered in order to understand the metabolic control of food intake. In general, integration could occur neurally, with separate sensors detecting changes in glucose and fat metabolism, or it could take place biochemically, with an event common to the metabolism of glucose and fat providing the signal. Elucidating the mechanism of integration requires that the nature of the metabolic signal(s) controlling feeding and the location of the receptor(s) detecting the signal(s) be identified. This chapter will deal with the issues of metabolic signal and receptor, starting first with the site of detection.

## II. A HEPATIC SIGNAL FOR AN INTEGRATED METABOLIC CONTROL OF FOOD INTAKE

Both brain and liver have been implicated in the detection of changes in fuel metabolism that control food intake.[1] There is evidence that glucose analogues (e.g., 2-deoxy-D-glucose or 5-thio-D-glucose), which inhibit glucose utilization and trigger feeding behavior, have both central and hepatic sites of action.[13-16] In contrast, agents that inhibit fatty acid oxidation (e.g., methyl palmoxirate and mercaptoacetate) appear to stimulate feeding by their action in the liver and other peripheral visceral tissues.[13,14,17,18] Using 2-deoxy-D-glucose to inhibit glucose utilization, Ritter and Taylor obtained evidence that signals for feeding generated by fatty acid and glucose metabolism arise from, respectively, peripheral and central sites, and that integration of this information therefore occurs neurally in the brain stem.[13] We have been studying the metabolic control of food intake using the fructose analogue, 2,5-anhydro-D-mannitol (2,5-AM), which triggers feeding by its action in liver.[19] The results of this work suggest that changes in both glucose and fatty acid metabolism are involved in the eating response to 2,5-AM, and thereby point to a role for the liver in the integrated metabolic control of food intake.

We initially examined 2,5-AM for its effect on food intake because it had been shown to have significant effects on liver metabolism and, as fructose does not cross the blood-brain barrier, was not expected to affect cerebral metabolism like glucose analogues do. In addition, we had found that administration of fructose reduced food intake by its action in liver.[20] 2,5-AM is metabolized like fructose to the mono- and then bisphosphate forms, but is not further metabolized through glycolysis.[21] Generally, its effect in liver is to "freeze" glucose metabolism by inhibiting glycogenolysis, gluconeogenesis, and glycolysis.[21-25] Our first experiments showed that intragastric or intraperitoneal administration of 2,5-AM elicited eating in rats in a dose-dependent manner.[26] The effect was not dependent on insulin and was accompanied by changes in plasma fuels indicative of a mild fast (i.e., slight drop in glucose and increase in fatty acids, glycerol, and ketone bodies).

The absence of any signs of behavioral impairment (ataxia) or unusual metabolic responses (e.g., hyperglycemia), which are indicative of a cerebral energetic emergency, and are often seen after administration of glucose analogues, suggested that 2,5-AM had a peripheral site of action. Results from subsequent experiments[19] provide direct evidence that 2,5-AM acts in liver to trigger eating:

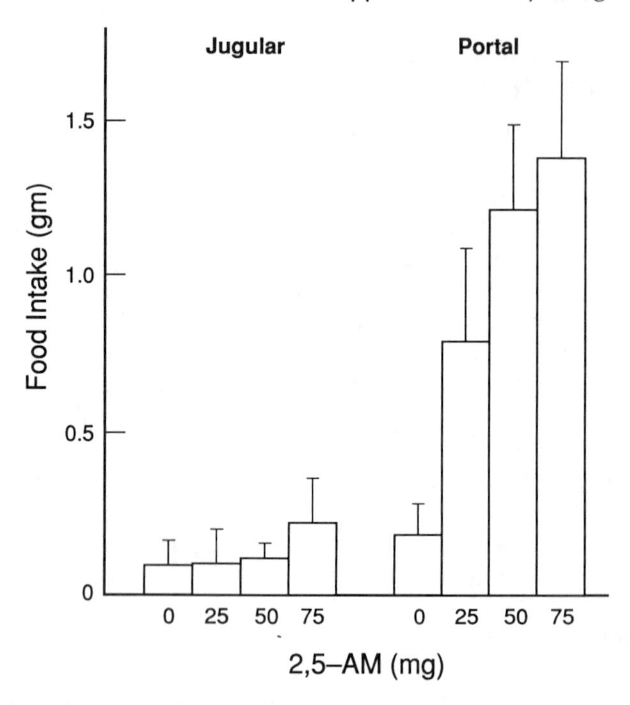


**FIGURE 2.** 2,5-anhydro-D-mannitol (2,5-AM) elicits feeding behavior in rats by its action in liver. Rats were given different amounts of 2,5-AM either via the jugular vein or hepatic portal vein.[19] Data show intakes in first 30 min of infusion; dose of 2,5-AM is total amount infused during this period. Values are means ± SEM of 7 to 9 rats.

1. Hepatic portal vein infusions of 2,5-AM elicit feeding within 15 min (Figure 2), whereas jugular vein infusions are ineffective at low doses (50 mg/h) or elicit eating only after a 30 min delay at the highest dose tested (150 mg/h).
2. $^{14}C$-labeled 2,5-AM given orally is taken up mainly in liver, but is undetectable in brain.
3. Hepatic branch vagotomy abolishes the eating response to 2,5-AM.

These findings point to a hepatic site for a signal that triggers feeding in rats. To determine whether this signal was involved in an integrated metabolic control of feeding behavior, we examined the role of fatty acid metabolism in the eating response to 2,5-AM.

Previous research has shown that the effect of metabolic inhibitors on food intake depends on the availability of alternative fuels. Inhibition of fatty acid oxidation increases feeding when rats are fed a high-fat, low-carbohydrate diet, but not when they are fed a high-carbohydrate diet.[8,10,27] Conversely, feeding a high-fat diet reduces the eating response to inhibition of glucose

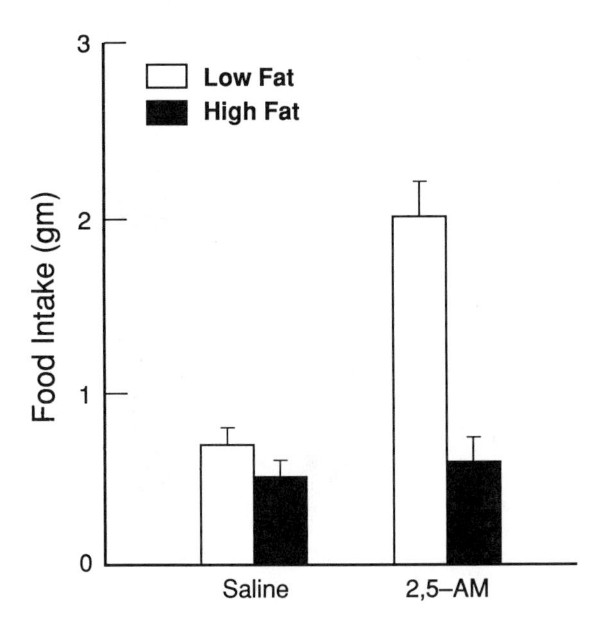


**FIGURE 3.** Feeding a high-fat diet prevents the eating response to 2,5-anhydro-D-mannitol (2,5-AM) in rats. Rats were maintained on a high-fat, low-carbohydrate (CHO) diet (63% of kcal from fat, 13% from CHO) or an isocaloric low-fat, high-CHO diet (13% of kcal from fat, 63% from CHO). Food intakes were measured 1 h after injection (i.p.) of 400 mg/kg 2,5-AM. Values are means ± SEM of 16 rats.

metabolism.[9] These interactions provide another line of evidence for an integrated metabolic control of feeding behavior by showing that the effect on feeding of inhibiting metabolism of one fuel can be offset by provision of an alternative fuel. Therefore, in one study we examined the effect of dietary fat and carbohydrate content on the eating response to 2,5-AM. As shown in Figure 3, the response to 2,5-AM was dependent on the dietary content of fat. Rats fed the low-fat diet increased food intake significantly in response to injection of 2,5-AM whereas those fed the high-fat diet did not.

To determine more directly whether feeding elicited by 2,5-AM depends on the status of fatty acid metabolism, we also examined the effects of combined treatment with 2,5-AM and methyl palmoxirate (MP; methyl 2-tetradecylglycidate), an inhibitor of fatty acid oxidation.[28] Rats were maintained on a high-fat, low-carbohydrate diet. As found previously,[8,29] MP alone increased feeding in rats fed this high-fat diet, whereas 2,5-AM alone did not. However, when both MP and 2,5-AM were administered, rats increased feeding in a synergistic fashion (Figure 4).

The high-fat diet used in these experiments has been shown to shift fat metabolism away from storage and towards oxidation,[30,31] whereas MP is

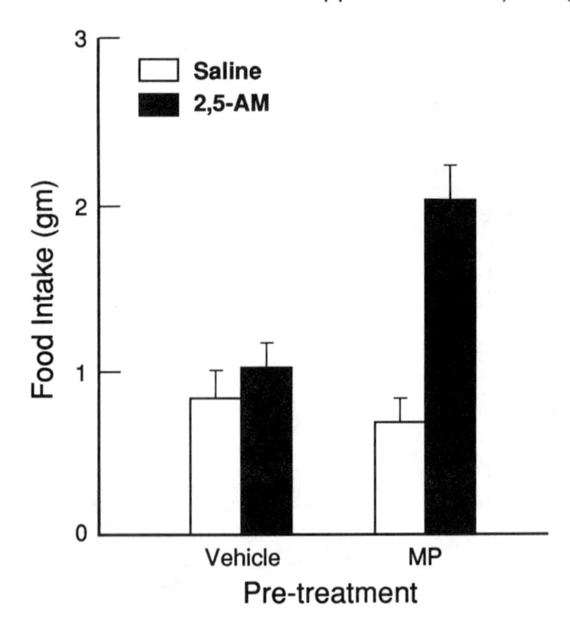


**FIGURE 4.** Synergistic increase in food intake of rats given combined treatment with methyl palmoxirate (MP) and 2,5-anhydro-D-mannitol (2,5-AM). Rats maintained on a high-fat, low-carbohydrate diet (63% of kcal from fat, 13% from CHO) were given 5 mg/kg methyl palmoxirate (MP) to inhibit fatty acid oxidation or its vehicle, followed 3 h later by injection (i.p.) of either 200 mg/kg 2,5-AM or saline. Food intake was measured 2 h after injection of 2,5-AM. Values are means ± SEM of 11 rats.

known to inhibit fatty acid oxidation.[28] Thus, these results indicate that the eating response to 2,5-AM is dependent (in an inverse manner) on the capacity to oxidize fatty acids; the response is enhanced when hepatic fatty acid oxidation is low and is prevented when it is high. Because the primary metabolic effect of 2,5-AM is inhibition of hepatic glucose metabolism, the results strongly suggest that the eating response to the analogue is triggered by a signal sensitive to the metabolism of both glucose and fatty acids. Because 2,5-AM elicits feeding by its action in liver,[19] and inhibition of fatty acid oxidation appears to trigger eating via a peripheral, perhaps hepatic, signal,[13,14,17,18] it is possible that this integrated signal has a hepatic origin.

## III. BIOCHEMISTRY OF THE HEPATIC SIGNAL FOR FEEDING

Given its pivotal role in the processing of glucose and fat fuels, and its importance in the disposition of fuels during both feeding and fasting, the liver is in a unique position to monitor changes in fuel metabolism that control eating behavior.[2] Russek was the first to propose such a role for the liver.[32] Since then, considerable evidence has accumulated indicating that changes in liver metabolism can restrain or terminate feeding behavior as well as initiate it.[1,33]

The nature of the hepatic signal controlling feeding behavior has not been elucidated. Russek[33] proposed a number of potential stimuli, including the level of liver glycogen, reducing sugars and pyruvate, but these suggestions lack experimental support. Insulin and glucagon have been implicated in the hepatic control of feeding,[34,35] but although they are thought to act via changes in hepatic metabolism, the metabolic signal has not been specified.

If changes in hepatic glucose and fatty acid metabolism interact to control feeding behavior, it is possible that a biochemical event common to the utilization of different metabolic fuels may provide a hepatic stimulus for eating. The notion that the metabolic stimulus for feeding behavior is a biochemical parameter common to metabolism of different fuels was first suggested by Kassil et al.[36] They proposed that food consumption was determined by the liberation of energy in food, and specifically by metabolites of the tricarboxylic acid (Krebs) cycle, although they did not indicate which metabolites provide the signal. Others have made a similar suggestion, emphasizing the Krebs cycle or the process of oxidative phosphorylation, without specifying the precise nature of the signal.[2,5,6] The hypothesis that a signal controlling feeding is generated by the liberation of energy from metabolic fuels is attractive because of its parsimony and its broad explanatory power.[37] However, despite its theoretical appeal, this hypothesis cannot be validated unless the stimulus can be identified.

Several investigators have proposed that a decrease in the level of adenosine triphosphate (ATP) is a metabolic stimulus triggering feeding behavior.[38,39] Because ATP is a final common product of the oxidation of both glucose and fatty acids, changes in the level of ATP in hepatocytes could provide an integrated signal for feeding behavior. However, ATP has not been measured to test its involvement in the control of feeding.

Localization of 2,5-AM's site of action to the liver and its known biochemical effects prompted us to focus first on this analogue as a tool to examine the role of ATP as a stimulus for feeding. *In vitro* studies with hepatocytes have shown that 2,5-AM decreases ATP.[25] 2,5-AM is treated like fructose through its first two steps of metabolism, in which it is phosphorylated in the C1 and then C6 position.[21] Rapid administration of fructose results in a transient decrease in ATP[40,41] because the rapid phosphorylation of fructose traps inorganic phosphate ($P_i$) in the form of mono- and diphosphorylated intermediates.[40,41] The resulting low level of intracellular $P_i$ in turn limits phosphorylation of adenosine and the production of ATP. We have begun studies to determine whether 2,5-AM is phosphorylated and decreases ATP *in vivo* under conditions in which it elicits feeding behavior,

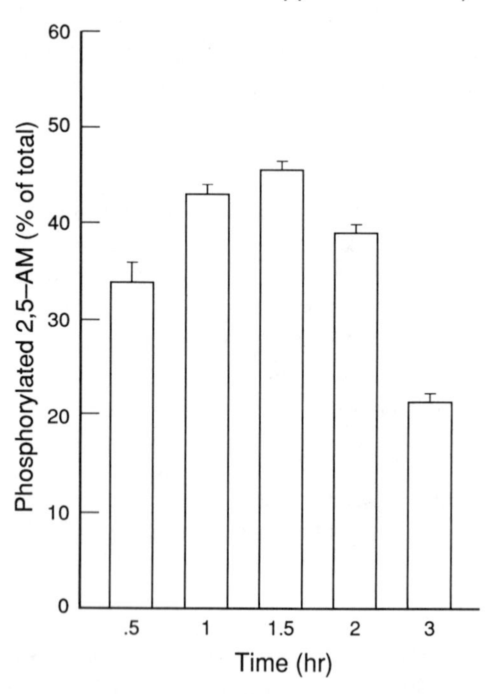


**FIGURE 5.** Phosphorylation of 2,5-anhydro-D-mannitol (2,5-AM) in rat liver. Livers taken from rats at various times after administration (p.o.) of 200 mg/kg containing 4.5 μCi/kg uniformly labeled 2,5-[$^{14}$C]AM. Tissue extracts were analyzed using thin-layer chromatography. Data are displayed as percent of total 2,5-AM that was phosphorylated. Values are means ± SEM of 4 rats per time point.

and whether phosphate trapping plays a role in the metabolic and behavioral effects of the analogue.

Thin-layer chromatography of liver extracts from rats given radiolabeled 2,5-AM showed that 2,5-AM is phosphorylated in liver by 30 min after oral administration. The proportion of phosphorylated to nonphosphorylated 2,5-AM increased over time to 50% by 90 min postadministration and then fell thereafter (Figure 5). The time course of phosphorylation of 2,5-AM thus parallels its effect on food intake because the eating response usually occurs between 60 and 90 min after intragastric administration. This is consistent with a role for 2,5-AM phosphorylation in the analogue's effect on food intake.

Reduced levels of ATP result in increased concentrations of adenosine diphosphate and adenosine monophosphate (AMP). A decrease in ATP, as well as in $P_i$, increases the activity of enzymes that degrade AMP to inosine, which is then converted to uric acid. Uric acid levels in blood and urine of rats increase after fructose loading, which depletes ATP and $P_i$.[42] Excretion

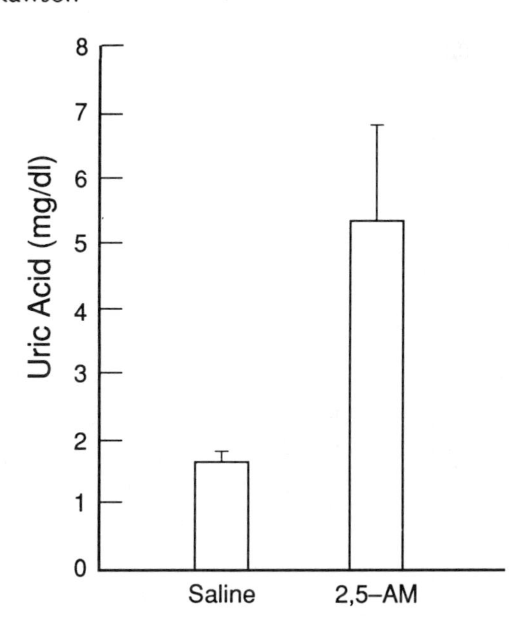


**FIGURE 6.** 2,5-Anhydro-D-mannitol (2,5-AM) increases urinary uric acid excretion in rats. Urine was collected for 2 h after injection (i.p.) with 200 mg/kg 2,5-AM or saline. Values are means ± SEM of 5 rats.

of uric acid in urine also increases in rats by 2 h after injection of 2,5-AM (Figure 6). This result indicates that 2,5-AM depletes ATP and $P_i$ when administered *in vivo*, and is consistent with the possibility that a decrease in hepatic ATP triggers the feeding response to the analogue.

To more directly assess the effect of 2,5-AM on hepatic ATP and $P_i$, we have employed $^{31}P$ nuclear magnetic resonance spectroscopy (NMRS).[43] These experiments were conducted in anesthetized animals using a Helmholtz nuclear magnetic resonance coil placed in contact with the liver. Analysis of spectra collected during intravenous infusion of 2,5-AM revealed decreases in ATP (Figure 7) and $P_i$, accompanied by an increase in phosphomonoesters, which, as shown by high-resolution NMRS of liver extracts, are comprised mostly of phosphorylated 2,5-AM. These changes became apparent after 30 min of infusion, which corresponds to the time at which food intake increases with this dose and route of administration in conscious animals. The results are consistent with the proposal that 2,5-AM decreases ATP by trapping phosphate.

A role for phosphate trapping in the behavioral response to 2,5-AM is further supported by the observation that injection of sodium phosphate prevents the feeding induced by 2,5-AM (Figure 8). Sodium chloride has no effect on the eating response, suggesting that the effect

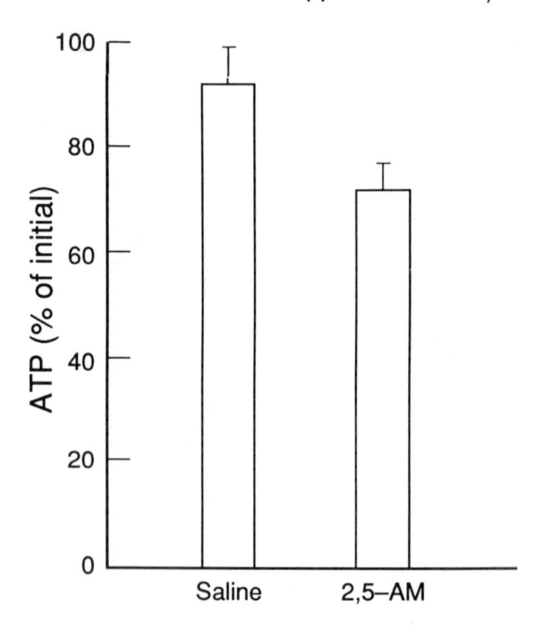


**FIGURE 7.** 2,5-Anhydro-D-mannitol (2,5-AM) decreases hepatic adenosine triphosphate *in vivo*. Anesthetized rats were infused (i.v.) with saline ($n = 3$) or 150 mg/kg 2,5-AM ($n = 6$) over 1 h while $^{31}P$ nuclear magnetic resonance spectroscopy was performed on their livers. Data shown are percent of initial ATP level at 75 min after the start of infusion. Values are means ± SEM.

is specific to the phosphate anion. Sodium phosphate injection does not affect the eating response to acute insulin treatment, and phosphate injection does not increase water intake during the period it prevents the eating response to 2,5-AM. These results indicate that the effect of phosphate injection is behaviorally specific; that is, the effect on the eating response to 2,5-AM is not due to malaise or elicitation of competing behaviors.

These results provide the first direct evidence that a decrease in ATP provides a signal to initiate feeding behavior. It seems unlikely that decreased $P_i$ is the signal to eat because $P_i$ in liver increases during fasting[44,45] when the need to eat is high. Rather, it seems more likely a reduction in $P_i$ due to phosphorylation of 2,5-AM decreases ATP production, which then provides a stimulus to eat. Accordingly, even though a decrease in ATP may trigger feeding, changes in phosphate availability would not be expected to play a part in the initiation of feeding under all circumstances (e.g., insulin-induced eating). Whether there are situations in which disturbances in phosphate metabolism produce changes in food intake remain to be seen.

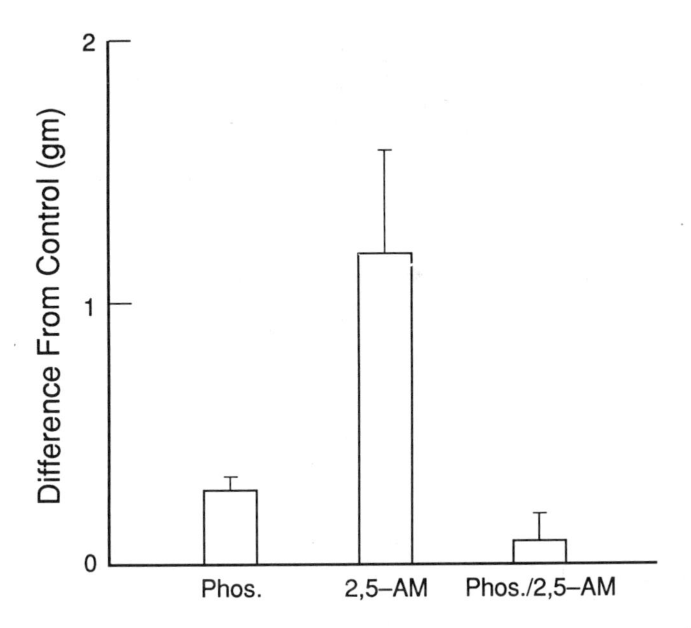


**FIGURE 8.** Phosphate loading prevents the eating response to 2,5-anhydro-D-mannitol (2,5-AM). Rats were injected (i.p.) with 0.91 mmol/kg of sodium chloride or sodium phosphate followed 5 min later by injection (i.p.) of saline or 300 mg/kg 2,5-AM. Data are shown as difference in 2 h food intake from that observed after treatment with sodium chloride and saline. Values are means ± SEM of 8 rats.

## IV. SUMMARY AND CONCLUSIONS

The results described above point to a mechanism for the control of feeding that integrates information from changes in peripheral glucose and fatty acid metabolism. The liver is apparently involved in this integrative control, but the nature of its role is unclear because the mechanism of integration remains unresolved. It is possible that separate signals associated with glucose and fatty acid metabolism arise in the liver or other peripheral tissues and are then integrated in the brain. Alternatively, changes in glucose and fatty acid metabolism may be integrated biochemically in the liver. Our findings implicating decreased hepatic ATP as a signal for feeding supports this interpretation because ATP production is a final common pathway in the metabolism of both glucose and fatty acids.

In the effort to elucidate the metabolic control of feeding behavior we are faced with the fundamental problems in sensory physiology of identifying the receptor and the stimulus. Identification of the liver as a site of action of experimental treatments that affect food intake via an integrative mechanism of control is an important step because it provides a starting point for an analysis of the metabolic and neural mechanisms of feeding behavior. This analysis is further facilitated by the focus on initiation of feeding or increases in eating behavior because elicitation or enhancement of behavior is more easily interpreted than decreases in behavior, which can be due to nonspecific effects of experimental treatments. However, further characterization of the metabolic stimulus in liver that initiates feeding will undoubtedly provide important insights into metabolic mechanisms of satiety as well.

## ACKNOWLEDGMENTS

This work was supported by NIH Grants DK-36339 and DC-00014 and by a grant from the Howard Heinz Endowment.

## REFERENCES

1. Friedman, M. I., Making sense out of calories. In: *Handbook of Behavioral Neurobiology: Food and Water Intake,* E. M. Stricker, Ed. Plenum, New York, 1990, 513.
2. Friedman, M. I., and Stricker, E. M., The physiological psychology of hunger: a physiological perspective, *Psychol. Rev.,* 83, 409, 1976.
3. Le Magnen, J., Devos, M., Gaudilliere, J.-P., Louis-Sylvestre, J., and Tallon, S., Role of a lipostatic mechanism in regulation by feeding of energy balance in rats, *J. Comp. Physiol. Psychol.,* 84, 1, 1973.
4. Mayer, J., Regulation of energy intake and the bodyweight: the glucostatic theory and the lipostatic hypothesis, *Ann. N.Y. Acad. Sci.,* 63,15, 1955.
5. Booth, D. A., Postabsorptively induced suppression of appetite and the energostatic control of feeding, *Physiol. Behav.,* 9, 199, 1972.
6. Panksepp, J., Effects of fats, proteins, and carbohydrates on food intake in rats, *Psychon. Monogr. Suppl.,* 4, 86, 1971.
7. Friedman, M. I., Hyperphagia in rats with experimental diabetes mellitus: a response to a decreased supply of utilizable fuels, *J. Comp. Physiol. Psychol.,* 92, 109, 1978.
8. Friedman, M. I., Tordoff, M. G., and Ramirez, I., Integrated metabolic control of food intake, *Brain Res. Bull.,* 17, 855, 1986.
9. Tordoff, M. G., Flynn, F. W., Grill, H. J., and Friedman, M. I., Contribution of fat metabolism to "glucoprivic" feeding produced by fourth ventricular 5-thio-D-glucose, *Brain Res.,* 445, 216, 1988.
10. Friedman, M. I., and Tordoff, M. G., Fatty acid oxidation and glucose utilization interact to control food intake in rats, *Am. J. Physiol.,* 251, R840, 1986.
11. Even, P. C., Coulaud, H., and Nicolaidis, S., Integrated metabolic control of food intake after 2-deoxy-D-glucose and nicotinic acid injection, *Am. J. Physiol.,* 255, R82, 1988.

12. Coscina, D. V., Synergism of 2-deoxyglucose and methyl palmoxirate on feeding but not metabolism, *Int. J. Obes.,* 15(Suppl. 3), 27, 1991.
13. Ritter, S., and Taylor, J. S., Capsaicin abolishes lipoprivic but not glucoprivic feeding in rats, *Am. J. Physiol.,* 256, R1232, 1989.
14. Ritter, S., and Taylor, J. S., Vagal sensory neurons are required for lipoprivic but not glucoprivic feeding in rats, *Am. J. Physiol.,* 258, R1395, 1990.
15. Novin, D., VanderWeele, D. A., and Rezek, M., Infusion of 2-deoxy-D-glucose into the hepatic-portal system causes eating: evidence for peripheral glucoreceptors, *Science,* 181, 858, 1973.
16. Delprete, E., and Scharrer, E., Hepatic branch vagotomy attenuates the feeding response to 2-deoxy-D-glucose in rats, *Exp. Physiol.,* 75, 259, 1990.
17. Langhans, W., and Scharrer, E., Evidence for a vagally mediated satiety signal derived from hepatic fatty acid oxidation, *J. Autonom. Nerv. Sys.,* 18, 13, 1987.
18. Beverly, J. L., and Martin, R. J., Influence of fatty acid oxidation in lateral hypothalamus on food intake and body composition, *Am. J. Physiol.,* 261, R339, 1991.
19. Tordoff, M. G., Rawson, N., and Friedman, M. I., 2,5-Anhydro-D-mannitol acts in liver to initiate feeding, *Am. J. Physiol.,* 261, R283, 1991.
20. Tordoff, M. G., and Friedman, M. I., Hepatic control of feeding: effect of glucose, fructose, and mannitol infusion, *Am. J. Physiol.,* 254, R969, 1988.
21. Riquelme, P. T., Kneer, N. M., Wernette-Hammond, M. E., and Lardy, H. A., Inhibition by 2,5-anhydro-D-mannitol of glycolysis in isolated rat hepatocytes and Ehrlich ascites cells, *Proc. Natl. Acad. Sci. U.S.A.*, 82, 78 1985.
22. Riquelme, P. T., Wernette-Hammond, M. E., Kneer, N. M., and Lardy, H. A., Regulation of carbohydrate metabolism by 2,5-anhydro-D-mannitol, *Proc. Natl. Acad. Sci. U.S.A.,* 80, 4301, 1983.
23. Riquelme, P. T., Wernette-Hammond, M. E., Kneer, N. M., and Lardy, H. A., Mechanism of action of 2,5-anhydro-D-mannitol in hepatocytes, *J. Biol. Chem.,* 259, 5115, 1984.
24. Hanson, R. L., Ho, R. S., Wisenberg, J. J., Simpson, R., Younathan, E. S., and Blair, J. B., Inhibition of gluconeogenesis and glycogenolysis by 2,5-anhydro-D-mannitol, *J. Biol. Chem.,* 259, 218, 1984.
25. Stevens, H. C., Covey, T. R., and Dills, W. L., Jr., Inhibition of gluconeogenesis by 2,5-anhydro-D-mannitol in isolated rat hepatocytes, *Biochim. Biophys. Acta,* 845, 506, 1985.
26. Tordoff, M. G., Rafka, R., DiNovi, M. J., and Friedman, M. I., 2,-5-Anhydro-D-mannitol: a fructose analogue that increases food intake in rats, *Am. J. Physiol.,* 254, R150, 1988.
27. Scharrer, E., and Langhans, W., Control of food intake by fatty acid oxidation, *Am. J. Physiol.,* 250, R1003, 1986.
28. Tutwiler, G. F., Ho, W., and Mohrbacher, R. J., 2-Tetradecylglycidic acid, *Methods Enzymol.,* 72, 533-551, 1981.
29. Friedman, M. I., Ramirez, I., Bowden, C. R., and Tordoff, M. G., Fuel partitioning and food intake: role for mitochondrial fatty acid transport, *Am. J. Physiol.,* 258, R216, 1990.
30. Ramirez, I., and Friedman, M. I., Dietary hyperphagia in rats: role of fat, carbohydrate and energy content, *Physiol. Behav.,* 47, 1157, 1990.

31. Reed, D. R., Tordoff, M. G., and Friedman, M. I., Enhanced acceptance and metabolism of fats by rats fed a high-fat diet, *Am. J. Physiol.*, 261, R1084, 1991.
32. Russek, M., Participation of hepatic glucoreceptors in the control of intake of food, *Nature (London)*, 197, 79, 1963.
33. Russek, M., Current status of the heptostatic theory of food intake control, *Appetite*, 2, 137, 1981.
34. Oetting, R. L., and VanderWeele, D. A., Insulin suppresses intake without inducing illness in sham feeding rats, *Physiol. Behav.*, 34, 557, 1985.
35. Le Sauter, J., Noh, U., and Geary, N., Hepatic portal infusion of glucagon antibodies increases spontaneous meal size in rats, *Am. J. Physiol.*, 261, R162, 1991.
36. Kassil, V. G., Ugolev, A. M., and Chernigovskii, V. N., Regulation of selection and consumption of food and metabolism, *Prog. Physiol. Sci.*, 1, 387, 1970.
37. Friedman, M. I., Metabolic control of calorie intake. In: *Chemical Senses, Volume 4: Appetite and Nutrition*, M. I. Friedman, M. G. Tordoff, and M. R. Kare, Eds. Marcel Dekker, New York, 1991, 19.
38. Scharrer, E., and Langhans, W., Mechanisms for the effect of body fat on food intake. In: *The Control of Body Fat Content*, J. M. Forbes, and G. R. Hervey, Eds. Smith-Gordon, London, 1990, 63.
39. Nicolaidis, S., and Even, P. C., The ischymetric control of feeding, *Int. J. Obes.*, 14(Suppl. 3), 35, 1990.
40. Burch, H. B., Lowry, O. H., Meinhardt, L., Max, P., Jr., and Chyu, K.-J., Effect of fructose, dihydroxyacetone, glycerol, and glucose on metabolites and related compounds in liver and kidney, *J. Biol. Chem.*, 245, 2092, 1970.
41. Morris, R. C., Nigon, K., and Reed, E. B., Evidence that the severity of depletion of inorganic phosphate determines the severity of the disturbance of adenine nucleotide metabolism in the liver and renal cortex of the fructose-loaded rat, *J. Clin. Invest.*, 61, 209, 1978.
42. Van den Berghe, G., Bronfman, M., Vanneste, R., and Hers, H.-G., The mechanism of adenosine triphosphate depletion in the liver after a load of fructose, *Biochem. J.*, 162, 20, 1977.
43. Rawson, N. E., Blum, H., Osbakken, M. D., and Friedman, M. I., Hepatic phosphate trapping, decreased ATP and increased feeding after 2,5-anhydro-*D*-mannitol. *Am. J. Physiol.*, in press.
44. Cunningham, C. C., Malloy, C. R., and Radda, G. K., Effect of fasting and acute ethanol administration on the energy state of in vivo liver as measured by $^{31}$P-NMR spectroscopy, *Biochim. Biophys. Acta*, 885, 12, 1986.
45. Desmoulin, F., Cozzone, P. J., and Canioni, P., Phosphorus-31 nuclear-magnetic-resonance study of phosphorylated metabolites compartmentation, intracellular pH and phosphorylation state during normoxia, hypoxia and ethanol perfusion in the perfused rat liver, *Eur. J. Biochem.*, 162, 151, 1987.

# 6 Neural Substrates for Metabolic Controls of Feeding

**Sue Ritter and Noel Y. Calingasan**

Deficits in the metabolic availability of glucose and fatty acids are powerful stimuli for initiation of feeding. The relationship between meal initiation and decreased availability of specific metabolic fuels can be demonstrated experimentally by administration of antimetabolic drugs that interfere with fuel utilization. 2-Deoxy-D-glucose (2DG) and 2-mercaptoacetate (MA) are examples of antimetabolic drugs that have been particularly useful in studying metabolic control of feeding, and are the major antimetabolic agents used in the work described in this chapter. 2-Deoxy-D-glucose causes glucoprivation by competitive blockade of phosphohexose-isomerase.[1,2] Mercaptoacetate causes lipoprivation by blocking mitochondrial acyl-CoA-dehydrogenases, thereby reducing β-oxidation of fatty acids.[3]

Because neither the precise location of the metabolic receptor cells that monitor fuel availability nor the metabolic step that serves as the transduction signal for stimulation of feeding by glucoprivic or lipoprivic agents is known, the extent to which these controls may converge on a common metabolic event is unclear. However, anatomical studies summarized in this chapter provide strong support for the hypothesis that 2DG and MA stimulate feeding by activating neural pathways that are at least partially separate.[9]

## I. LIPOPRIVIC FEEDING

### A. Dependence on Vagal Sensory Neurons

Several lines of investigation indicate that decreased fatty acid availability is detected peripherally and that vagal sensory neurons play an essential role in the afferent transmission of the sensory message eventually leading to the stimulation of food intake. Although it is not yet known whether vagal

0-8493-4466-2/94/$0.00+$.50

sensory neurons are themselves the metabolic receptors, or whether these neurons innervate metabolic receptor cells of other sorts, their crucial role in the stimulation of feeding has been revealed in surgical and chemical lesioning experiments and in studies of gene expression during metabolic challenge.

### 1. Surgical and Chemical Lesions

Evidence demonstrating the crucial role of vagal sensory neurons in lipoprivic feeding comes in part from chemical and surgical vagotomy experiments. Total subdiaphragmatic vagotomy by surgical transection of the two vagal trunks abolishes lipoprivic feeding, while the same animals continue to eat in response to 2DG (Figure 1).[10] Studies of lipoprivic feeding in rats with selective lesions of specific vagal branches[9,11] have indicated that fibers important for lipoprivic feeding are distributed in several, possibly all, subdiaphragmatic vagal branches. The majority, however, appear to travel in the gastric branches. Selective transection of the gastric vagal branches totally and permanently abolishes lipoprivic feeding (Figure 2). Transection of other vagal branches, singly or in various combinations, also impairs lipoprivic feeding (Figure 3), but these deficits are temporary. It is noteworthy that neither hepatic branch vagotomy nor total liver denervation abolished lipoprivic feeding in our experiments. Therefore, despite the presence of metabolically-sensitive fibers in the hepatic vagal branch[12-14] and previous data implicating this branch in lipoprivic feeding,[15] our data indicate that the hepatic branch per se is neither necessary nor sufficient for lipoprivic feeding.

The importance of vagal sensory neurons, as opposed to vagal motor neurons, in lipoprivic feeding has been demonstrated by the use of capsaicin. Capsaicin is a neurotoxin known to damage a subpopulation of primary sensory neurons possessing small diameter unmyelinated processes,[16,17] including many vagal sensory neurons,[18,19] while leaving motor neurons intact.[20] Systemic administration of capsaicin to adult rats permanently abolishes feeding induced by MA, but does not impair feeding induced by 2DG (Figure 4).[21] The role of vagal sensory neurons in lipoprivic feeding is further demonstrated in rats with aspiration lesions of central vagal sensory terminals in the area postrema and nucleus of the solitary tract (AP/NTS). Lesions of the AP/NTS that do not destroy the dorsal motor nucleus of the vagus also abolish lipoprivic feeding (Figure 4).[10] However, unlike capsaicin, AP/NTS lesions also impair glucoprivic feeding (see Section II.A).

The fact that vagal sensory neurons involved in lipoprivic feeding are not confined to a single vagal branch will increase the difficulty of locating specific sites or tissues where metabolic monitoring takes place. Distribution of the crucial fibers in multiple branches may indicate that receptors for lipoprivic feeding are in fact diffusely distributed in the abdominal viscera.

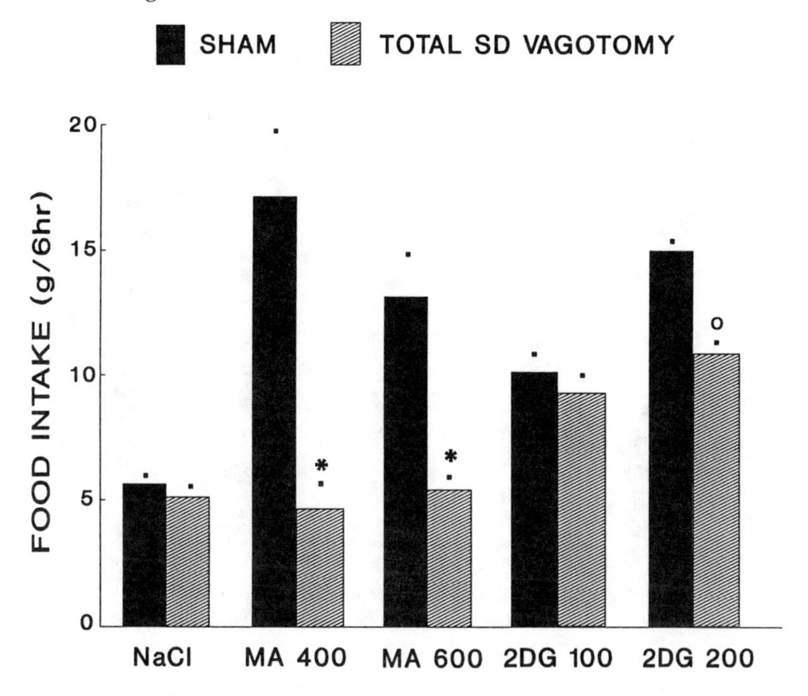


**FIGURE 1.** Food intake of subdiaphragmatic vagotomized rats and controls during 6-h tests after injection of NaCl (0.9%, mean of 4 tests), MA (400 and 600 μmol/kg, i.p.), and 2DG (100 and 200 mg/kg, s.c.). Rats were maintained and tested on a medium-fat, semi-solid diet. Means and standard errors (squares above bars) are shown. $^{*}p < 0.001$, lesion vs. sham; $^{\circ}p < 0.05$, lesion vs. sham.

Alternatively, these receptors may be located in a single abdominal site, such as the upper duodenum and pylorus, which is jointly innervated by several vagal branches.[22]

## 2. Neurochemical Approaches

Neurochemical approaches may provide a means of identifying the specific subpopulation(s) of vagal sensory neurons important for lipoprivic feeding. We have recently shown in rats that cell bodies of vagal sensory neurons in the nodose ganglion exhibit galanin-like immunoreactivity and express hybridizable galanin mRNA.[23] Since galanin is present in rat vagal sensory neurons and stimulates feeding,[24] particularly the intake of fat,[25,26] when injected intracranially in rats, it seems possible that vagal galanin may be a mediator of lipoprivic feeding. Therefore, we examined the effect of MA-induced lipoprivation on galanin mRNA expression in nodose ganglion cells using *in situ* hybridization with a well-characterized oligonucleotide probe complementary to nucleotides 259 to 303 of rat preprogalanin mRNA.[27]

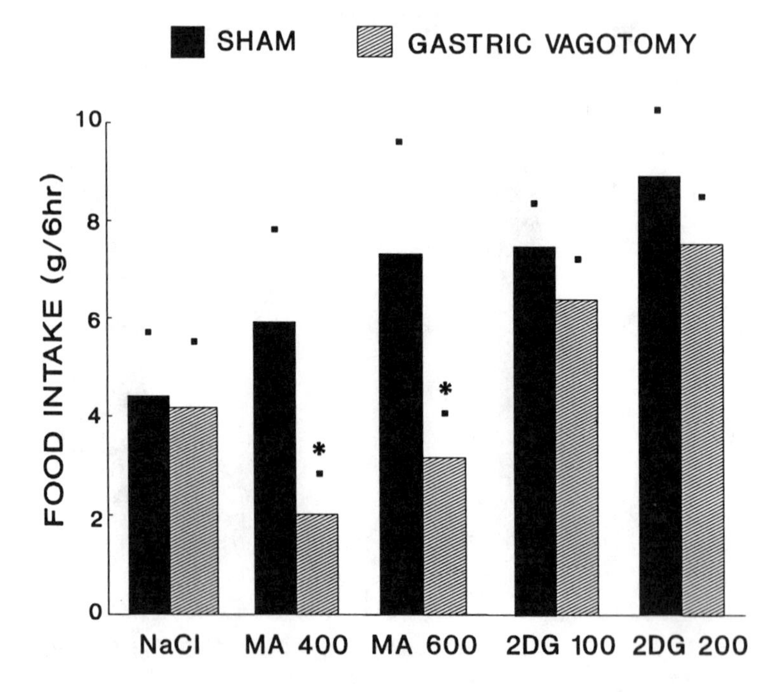


**FIGURE 2.** Food intake of rats with bilateral vagal gastric branch transections or sham vagotomies in a 6-h test following injection of saline (0.9%), MA (400 and 600 μmol/kg, i.p.), and 2DG (100 and 200 mg/kg, s.c.). Rats were maintained and tested on a medium-fat, semisolid diet. Means ± standard errors (squares above bars) are shown. $*p < 0.001$, lesion vs. sham.

Preliminary results show that MA, but not 2DG, cholecystokinin (CCK), or vehicle treatment significantly increases the number of nodose cell bodies containing hybridizable substrate. Thus, galanin may be a mediator of vagally elicited responses to lipoprivation, perhaps including lipoprivic feeding. The fact that the number of nodose cell bodies expressing galanin mRNA is not increased by CCK, a peptide that also requires vagal sensory neurons for its behavioral effect,[28,29] may indicate that galanin-containing vagal neurons are selectively sensitive to metabolic stimuli. Additional work is underway to test role of galanin in lipoprivic feeding.

## B. Central Neural Pathways

### 1. Lesion Studies

In one line of investigation we have combined brain lesions with behavioral studies to identify brain sites potentially involved in glucoprivic and lipoprivic feeding.[9,30] Our strategy in selecting central lesion sites was based in part on the fact that AP/NTS lesions severely impair both glucoprivic and

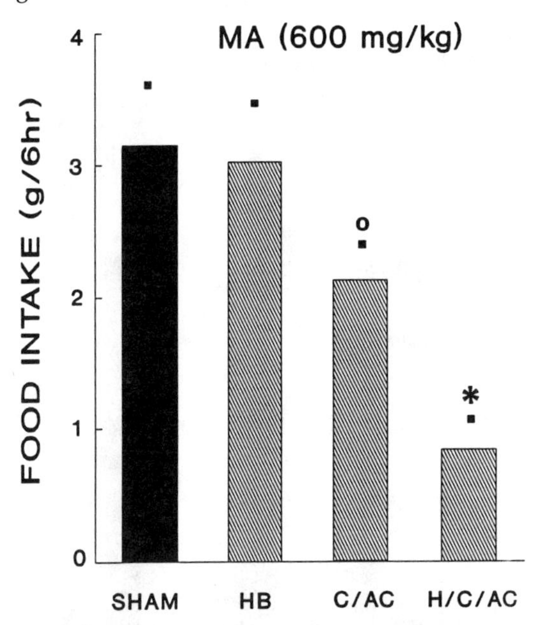


**FIGURE 3.** Intake of a medium-fat diet in a 6-h test after MA (600 μmol/kg, i.p.) in rats prepared 3 weeks prior to the start of testing by sham vagotomy (SHAM), hepatic vagalbranch (HB) transection, transection of the celiac and accessory celiac (C/AC) vagal branches, or transection of all three of these branches (H/C/AC). Means ± standard errors (squares above bars) are shown. **p* <0.001, lesion vs. sham; °*p* <0.05, lesion vs. sham.

lipoprivic feeding. These lesions destroy central terminals of vagal sensory neurons known to be important for lipoprivic feeding[10,21] and there is some evidence to suggest that this same lesion destroys actual receptor cells important for glucoprivic feeding (see Section II.A). Given its importance for both glucoprivic and lipoprivic feeding, the AP/NTS was our starting point for tracing the neural pathways for these controls more rostrally in the brain. In these studies, we placed electrolytic lesions in areas known to be innervated by projections from the AP/NTS[31-34] and examined the effects of the lesions on MA- and 2DG-induced feeding.

Our studies so far have demonstrated that the lateral parabrachial nucleus (LPBN) and the central nucleus of the amygdala (CNA), both major recipients of visceral sensory projections from AP/NTS neurons, are crucial for MA-induced feeding (Figure 5). In the LPBN, the cell bodies important for MA-induced feeding appear to be localized in the region occupied by the dorsal and central LPBN subnuclei, since both electrolytic and excitotoxin (ibotenic acid) microlesions centered in this region abolished feeding in response to MA (Figures 6 and 7).[35] Fibers of passage important for MA-induced feeding appear to pass through the external and superior LPBN since electrolytic but not

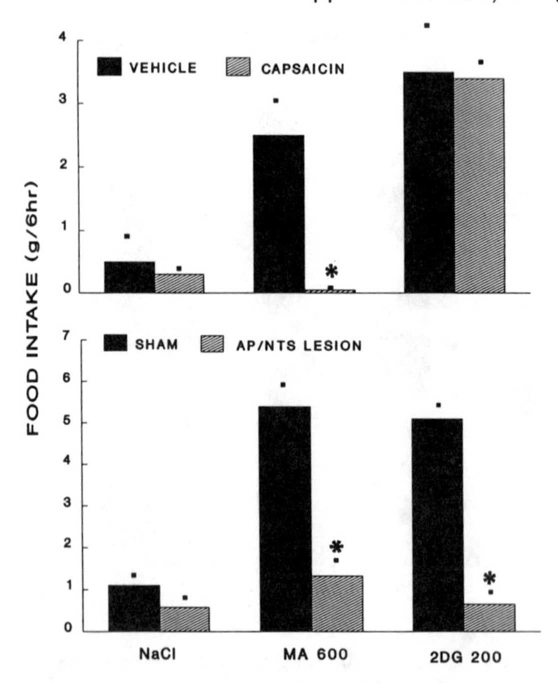


**FIGURE 4.** Cumulative food intake in a 6-h test after MA (600 μmol/kg), 2DG (200 mg/kg), or saline injection in rats with vagal sensory neuron lesions. Lesions were made by systemic injection of capsaicin (top panel) and by aspiration lesion of the AP/NTS (bottom panel). Control animals were injected with the capsaicin vehicle solution or given sham AP/NTS lesions, respectively. Feeding tests were conducted in undeprived rats during the light phase of circadian light cycle, using the animals' maintenance diet (a medium-fat powdered diet). Means ± standard errors (squares above bars) are shown. $*p < 0.001$, lesion vs. sham.

ibotenate lesions of these subnuclei disrupted the feeding response. The lPBN lesions caused deficits that were selective for MA-induced feeding and did not impair 2DG-induced feeding. Consistent with our findings, Flynn et al. have recently reported that LPBN lesions do not impair feeding induced by 2DG.[36]

Bilateral electrolytic destruction of the CNA also severely impaired or abolished MA-induced feeding. However, unlike lesions of the dorsal and central LPBN subnuclei, CNA lesions were not totally selective for MA-induced feeding. Feeding in response to 2DG was also impaired, especially at the lowest dose tested. Feeding in response to the higher 2DG dose was reduced compared to controls, but was not abolished. Impairment of feeding induced by low, but not high, 2DG doses in rats with CNA lesions was reported previously by Tordoff et al.[37]

The paraventricular nucleus of the hypothalamus (PVN) also receives a major projection from AP/NTS neurons. However, despite the importance

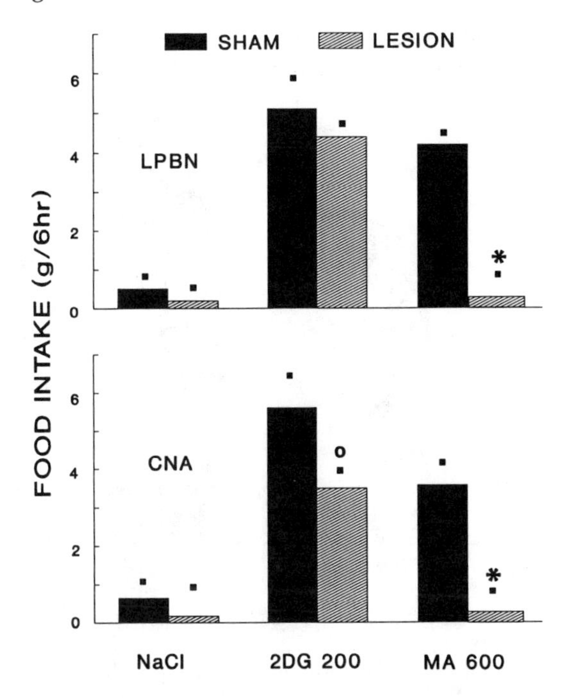


**FIGURE 5.** Intake of a medium-fat powdered diet by brain-lesioned rats and sham-operated controls in response to 2DG (200 mg/kg, s.c.) and MA (600 μmol/kg) and saline (NaCl, 0.9%). The top panel shows responses of rats with lesions destroying the entire lateral parabrachial nucleus (LPBN) bilaterally. The bottom panel shows responses of rats with lesions destroying the entire central nucleus of the amygdala (CNA) bilaterally. Means ± standard errors (squares above bars) are shown. *$p$ <0.001, lesion vs. sham; °$p$ <0.05, lesion vs. sham.

of the PVN for the control of food intake, total electrolytic destruction of the PVN did not impair either MA- or 2DG-induced feeding [38] in our study. Results showing that PVN lesions do not impair 2DG-induced feeding have been reported previously.[39]

## 2. Fos Immunohistochemistry

In a second series of studies, we used c-*fos* immunohistochemistry to identify neurons within the brain that are activated by systemic administration of 2DG and MA. Fos is the protein product of a proto oncogene (c-*fos)* that is induced in many neurons as an immediate-early response to activation. Fos protein, which can be detected by standard immunohistochemical techniques, increases in the nucleus of activated neurons beginning within minutes of stimulus presentation and has a half-life of about 2 h.[40]

We found that both MA and 2DG induce Fos-like immunoreactivity (Fos-li) in specific brain regions. The staining is remarkably specific and

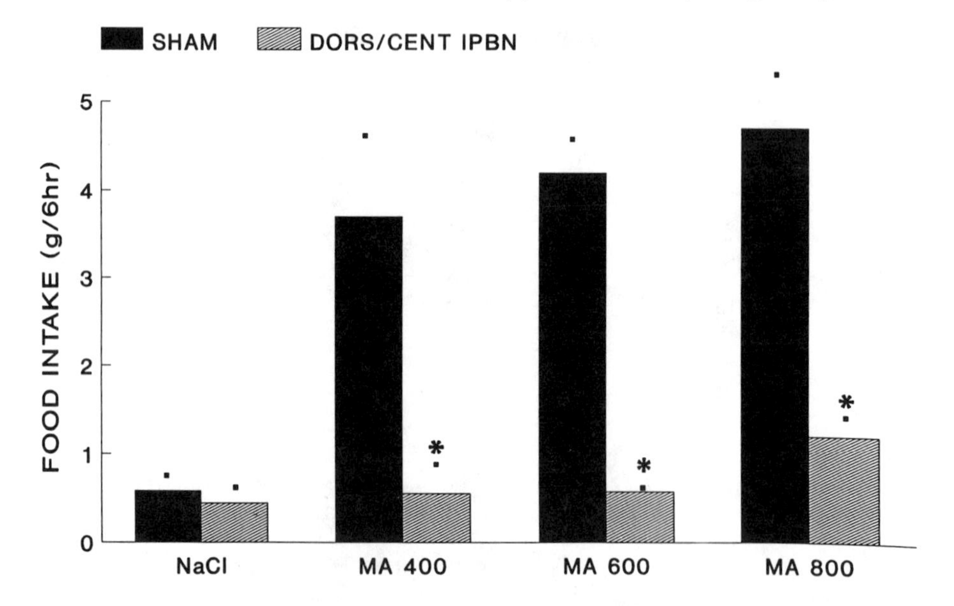


**FIGURE 6.** Cumulative food intake of rats with selective electrolytic lesions of the dorsal and central LPBN and sham-lesioned controls during 6-h tests after saline (NaCl, 0.9%, i.p.) or MA (400, 600, and 800 μmol/kg, i.p.). These lesions did not abolish 2DG-induced feeding. Means ± standard errors (squares above bars) are shown. *$p$ <0.001, lesion vs. sham.

reproducible for both drugs and is not induced by control injections. Effects of 2DG will be discussed in Section II.B. MA increases Fos-li markedly in the AP/NTS, the LPBN (central, dorsal, and external subnuclei), and CNA (lateral subnucleus) (Figure 8), and in the dorsal motor nucleus of the vagus. It is noteworthy that except for the vagal motor nucleus, the areas where MA increases Fos-li are the same areas where lesions cause deficits in MA-induced feeding. Similarly, it is noteworthy that MA is not an effective stimulus for induction of Fos-li in the PVN, a result that is consistent with the fact that PVN lesions do not impair MA-induced feeding.[38] Also consistent with results from feeding tests[10,21] was our finding that subdiaphragmatic vagotomy completely blocks induction of Fos-li by MA in all brain areas, but does not block induction of Fos-li by 2DG in the brain.

Together, c-*fos* and lesion results suggest that MA activates an afferent pathway that originates with vagal sensory neurons, projects with other higher order visceral sensory neurons from the AP/NTS to the LPBN and CNA, and ultimately innervates sites responsible for arousal of appetite in response to lipoprivation (Figure 9).

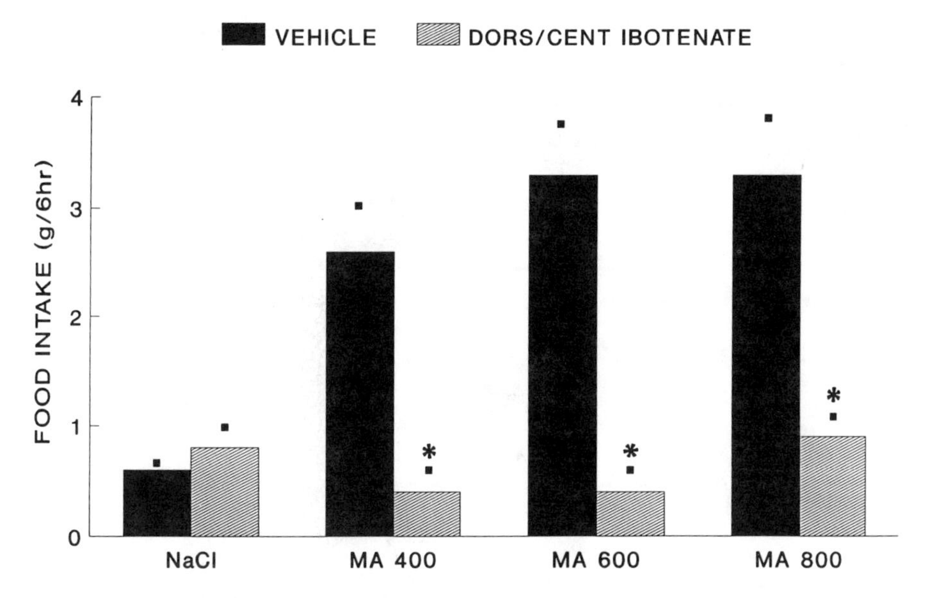


**FIGURE 7.** Cumulative food intake of rats with ibotenic acid lesions of the dorsal and central LPBN and vehicle-injected controls during 6-h tests after saline (NaCl, 0.9%, i.p.) or MA (400, 600, and 800 μmol/kg, i.p.). These lesions did not abolish 2DG-induced feeding. Lesions were confirmed using conventional cell stains and by analysis of the astrocytic scar as detected by immunohistochemical analysis of glial fibrillary acidic protein. *$p$ <0.001, lesion vs. sham.

## II. GLUCOPRIVIC FEEDING

### A. Evidence for Receptors within the Brain

Glucoprivic feeding is mediated by a population of metabolic receptors that appears to be different from those that mediate lipoprivic feeding. Unlike lipoprivic feeding, glucoprivic feeding does not require vagal sensory neurons,[10] is not capsaicin sensitive,[21] and can be stimulated by independent activation of metabolic receptors within the brain.[41-43]

The precise location of these central receptors for glucoprivic feeding is not yet known. However, convergent results from a number of experiments suggest that they may be located in the AP/NTS region. Cerebral aqueduct obstruction by injection of a silicone grease plug blocks the feeding response to lateral ventricular, but not fourth ventricular, injections of the glucoprivic agent 5-thioglucose. These results suggest that cells responsive to both lateral and fourth ventricular 5-thioglucose are located in the hindbrain caudal to the plug.[44] The possibility that this caudal site is the AP/NTS region is suggested by other studies showing that feeding in response to both central and systemic glucoprivation is severely impaired or abolished by AP/NTS lesions.[10,43,45,46]

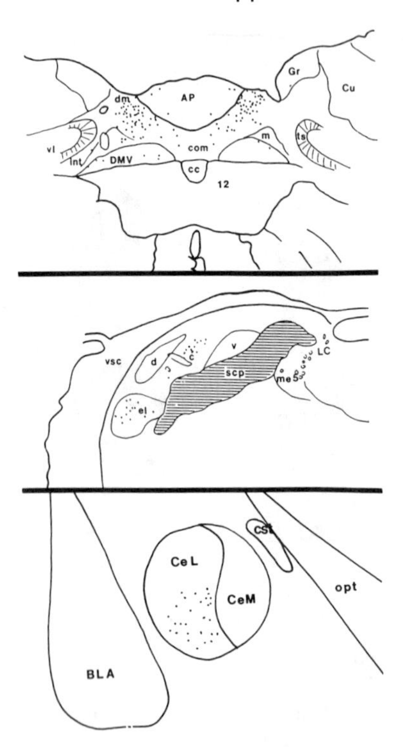


**FIGURE 8.** Camera lucida drawings (coronal plane) showing the distribution of Fos-li induced in rats by remote intravenous infusion of MA (600 μmol/kg) in the AP/NTS region (top panel), the dorsal and central LPBN subnuclei (middle panel), and the central subnucleus of the amygdala (CNA) (bottom panel). Fos-li was not induced in these areas by infusion of control solutions. Induction of Fos-li by MA in these brain areas was abolished by subdiaphragmatic vagotomy. Abbreviations (top panel): AP = area postrema; com, dm, int, m, and vl = commissural, dorsomedial, internal medial, and ventrolateral subnuclei of the nucleus of the solitary tract; cc = central canal; Cu = nucleus cuneatus; DMV = dorsal motor nucleus of the vagus; Gr = nucleus gracilis; ts = solitary tract; 12 = hypoglossal nucleus; (middle panel): c, d, el, v = central, dorsal, external lateral, and ventral subnuclei of the lateral parabrachial nucleus; LC = locus coeruleus; me5 = mesencephalic nucleus of the trigeminal nerve; scp = superior cerebellar peduncle; vsc = ventral spinocerebellar tract; (bottom panel): BLA = basolateral amygdaloid nucleus, anterior; CeL = central amygdaloid nucleus, lateral; CeM = central amygdaloid nucleus, medial; cst = commissural stria terminalis; opt = optic tract.

## B. Central Pathways

The central neural pathways mediating glucoprivic feeding are still largely unknown. However, it is clear from the lesion studies discussed above that glucoprivic feeding is mediated by central pathways other than or in addition to those responsible for lipoprivic feeding. Thus, the central

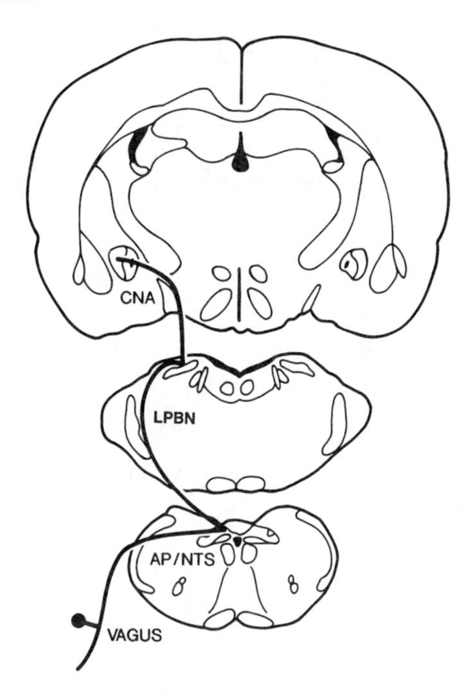


**FIGURE 9.** Schematic diagram depicting the putative afferent limb of the neural pathway responsible for lipoprivic feeding. Deficits in fatty acid oxidation are monitored in the abdominal viscera and related signals are transmitted to the brain by vagal sensory neurons that terminate in the AP/NTS region. Higher order neurons then transmit this information to the dorsal and/or central LPBN subnucleus and from there to the CNA (possibly the lateral subnucleus). Information ultimately reaches brain sites capable of initiating food intake. This putative pathway was delineated from behavioral studies of lipoprivic feeding in brain lesioned and vagotomized rats and from maps of Fos-li induced by systemic MA treatment.

neural pathways, as well as the receptor cells which monitor fuel utilization, are distinct for the two controls.

Whether Fos immunohistochemistry will be useful in delineating central pathways for glucoprivic feeding is still unclear. Mapping studies have revealed that 2DG induces Fos-li in the same areas where Fos-li is expressed in response to MA, but also in some areas where MA does not induce Fos-li. After 2DG administration, Fos-li is present in the AP/NTS, dorsal motor nucleus of the vagus, external LPBN subnucleus, dorsal and central LPBN, locus coeruleus, CNA, the the paraventricular nucleus of the thalamus, the supraoptic nucleus, and the PVN. Occasionally very light staining is present in the dorsal raphe. In contrast to MA, the ability of 2DG to induce Fos-li in these areas is not blocked by total subdiaphragmatic vagotomy. Thus,

2DG both induces Fos-li in the brain and stimulates food intake by vagally-independent mechanisms.

Although all of the areas expressing Fos-li in response to glucoprivation have not yet been examined for their role in glucoprivic feeding, lesion results discussed above indicate that many of these areas are not involved in or are not essential for the feeding response. Neurons expressing Fos-li in areas where lesions do not impair glucoprivic feeding may be involved in other responses to glucoprivation, such as sympathoadrenalmedullary activation,[47] though this remains to be determined. Furthermore, it is important to note that some areas, such as the dorsomedial and lateral hypothalamus, where excitotoxin lesions have been reported to produce deficits in glucoprivic feeding,[48,49] did not contain 2DG-induced Fos-li. Such results remind us of the possibility that neurons essential specifically for the feeding response to glucoprivation may not express c-*fos*.

### C. Peripheral Receptors

The existence of central glucoreceptors that are independently capable of stimulating feeding does not rule out a potential contribution of peripheral mechanisms to glucoprivic feeding. Several investigators have used subdiaphragmatic and selective hepatic branch vagotomies and other strategies in attempting to demonstrate such mechanisms.[50-55] However, past evidence for the existence of peripheral glucoreceptors controlling food intake, though in some cases tantalizing, has not been compelling.

Recently, the idea that peripheral glucoreceptors may contribute to the control of food intake has been invigorated by the findings of Tordoff and his colleagues.[56,57] These investigators have shown that feeding can be stimulated with the antimetabolic fructose analogue, 2,5-anhydro-D-mannitol (2,5-AM). Like fructose itself, this analogue does not appear to pass the blood-brain barrier and, therefore, its direct antimetabolic actions would be restricted to peripheral tissues and circumventricular organs. Rats begin eating sooner and eat more food during intraportal than during intrajugular infusions of 2,5-AM. Furthermore, the stimulation of feeding evoked by a low, but not a high, dose of 2,5-AM is blocked by hepatic vagotomy. The investigators have speculated that perhaps a role for peripheral (hepatic) mechanisms in stimulation of feeding by pharmacological impairment of carbohydrate metabolism is more clearly demonstrated with low 2,5-AM doses than with 2DG because the contribution of the peripheral mechanisms is not masked by the simultaneous activation of central receptors, as is the case with 2DG.

To further evaluate the role of the vagus in the response to high 2,5-AM doses, we have recently collaborated with Mark Friedman in assessing the ability of 2,5-AM (300 and 500 mg/kg) to induce Fos-li in the AP/NTS in sham-operated, hepatic branch vagotomized and total subdiaphragmatic vagotomized rats.[58] We found that both doses of 2,5-AM, but not equimolar doses of fructose, induce Fos-li in the AP/NTS. As with food intake, the effect of the lower but not the higher 2,5-AM dose on Fos-li is blocked by hepatic branch vagotomy. However, the high dose effect on Fos-li (and food intake) is blocked by total subdiaphragmatic vagotomy. These results are consistent with the hypothesis that stimulation of feeding by 2,5-AM, unlike 2DG-induced feeding, may be entirely dependent on the vagus. Hepatic branch neurons may have the lowest threshold for activation by 2,5-AM, while higher 2,5-AM doses stimulate neurons in other vagal branches.

It is tempting to speculate that peripheral receptors activated by 2,5-AM might be low threshold receptors positioned to detect local changes in carbohydrate availability (in the liver or elsewhere) that are not necessarily detectable in the systemic circulation.[56,57] Receptors with such a function could conceivably exert a glucoprivic control of meal initiation under conditions in which glucose deficits are not in evidence or in response to transient preprandial reductions similar to those reported by Louis-Sylvestre and LeMagnen[59] and Campfield et al.[60,61]

Experimental findings with 2,5-AM thus suggest that peripheral, as well as central, receptors contribute to the control of feeding by glucoprivation. It will be important to determine whether 2,5-AM activates a peripheral system that monitors carbohydrate metabolism selectively or whether receptors activated by 2,5-AM are the same receptors that monitor fatty acid oxidation. In other words, it will be important to determine whether integration of peripheral metabolic information occurs by convergence of signals from nutrient-specific systems onto a common population of higher order cells or by summation within a common population of receptors that is "multimodal" in its ability to respond to deficits in a variety of metabolic fuels.

## III. SUMMARY

In summary, we find that MA- and 2DG-induced feeding are neurologically different controls. The controls appear to be separable both at the level of signal detection and in their central projections. Specifically, 2DG stimulates feeding by activation of receptors within the brain, whereas MA-induced feeding is mediated by peripheral receptors and requires intact vagal sensory neurons. The central neural circuitry responsible for the hyperphagic effect of these two drugs is also different. Although the AP/NTS region is crucial for both 2DG- and MA-induced feeding, lesions of the LPBN abolish MA-induced feeding selectively. Thus, 2DG activates an extraparabrachial pathway for metabolic control of feeding that is not activated by MA. Though separate systems appear to be activated by 2DG and MA, experimental results are nevertheless clear in showing that the simultaneous activation of these distinct systems produces an integrated feeding response that takes into account the availability of both carbohydrates and fatty acids.[8,10,21] How and where this integration occurs, however, is not yet known.

## IV. CONCLUSION

The hypothesis that receptors for glucoprivic and lipoprivic feeding are located in the brain and abdominal viscera, respectively, has intuitive appeal. Brain cells use glucose, but not fatty acids, for energy metabolism and require uninterrupted delivery of glucose by the blood for survival. The localization in the brain itself of mechanisms to ensure its own glucose supply therefore seems reasonable. Similarly, it is reasonable that receptors monitoring fatty acid utilization would be located in peripheral tissues, for which fatty acids are an important metabolic substrate. The fact that systems responsive to deficits in fatty acid and glucose are distinct provides the opportunity for arousal of behavioral and physiological responses precisely tuned to specific and changing metabolic requirements. By understanding better how and where metabolic events are monitored, we can formulate stronger hypotheses about how these events might control food intake and metabolism.

## REFERENCES


1. Wick, A. N., Dury, D. R., Nakada, H. I., and Wolfe, J. B., Localization of the primary metabolic block produced by 2-deoxyglucose, *J. Biol. Chem.*, 224, 963, 1957.
2. Brown, J., Effects of 2-deoxy-D-glucose on carbohydrate metabolism: review of the literature and studies in the rat, *Metabolism*, 11, 1098, 1962.
3. Bauche, F., Sabourault, D., Giudicelli, Y., Nordmann, J., and Nordmann, R., Inhibition in vitro of acyl-CoA-dehydrogenases by 2-mercaptoacetate in rat liver mitochondria, *Biochem. J.*, 215, 457, 1983.
4. Smith, G. P., and Epstein, A. N., Increased feeding in response to decreased glucose utilization in the rat and monkey, *Am. J. Physiol.*, 217, 1083, 1969.
5. Epstein, A. N., Nicolaidis, S., and Miselis, R., The glucoprivic control of food intake and the glucostatic theory of feeding behavior. In: *Neural Integration of Physiological Mechanisms and Behavior*, G. J. Mogenson, and F. R. Calarescu, Eds. University Press, Toronto, 1975, 148.
6. Ritter, S., Glucoprivation and the glucoprivic control of food intake. In: *Food Intake: Neural and Humoral Controls*, R. C. Ritter, S. Ritter, and C. D. Barnes, Eds. Academic Press, Orlando, 1986, 268.
7. Scharrer, E., and Langhans, W., Control of food intake by fatty acid oxidation, *Am. J. Physiol.*, 250, R1003, 1986.
8. Friedman, M. I., Tordoff, M. G., and Ramirez, I., Integrated metabolic control of food intake, *Brain Res. Bull.*, 17, 855, 1986.

9. Ritter, S., Calingasan, N. Y., Hutton, B., and Dinh, T. T., Cooperation of vagal and central neural systems in monitoring metabolic events controlling feeding behavior. In: *Neuroanatomy and Physiology of Abdominal Vagal Afferents,* S. Ritter, R. C. Ritter, and C. D. Barnes, Eds. CRC Press, Boca Raton, FL, 1992, 249.
10. Ritter, S., and Taylor, J. S., Vagal sensory neurons are required for lipoprivic but not glucoprivic feeding in rats, *Am. J. Physiol.,* 258, R1395, 1990.
11. Ritter, S., Hutton, B. W., and Dinh, T. T., Neurons required for lipoprivic feeding are not limited to a single vagal branch, *Neurosci. Abstr.,* 16, 295, 1990.
12. Niijima, A., Glucose sensitive afferent nerve fibers in the liver and regulation of blood glucose, *Brain Res. Bull.,* 5 (Suppl. 4), 175, 1980.
13. Niijima, A., Suppression of afferent activity of the hepatic vagus nerve by anomers of D-glucose, *Am. J. Physiol.,* 244, R611, 1983.
14. Niijima, A., Nervous regulation of metabolism, *Prog. Neurobiol.,* 33, 135, 1989.
15. Langhans, W., and Scharrer, E., Evidence for a vagally mediated satiety signal derived from hepatic fatty acid oxidation, *J. Autonom. Nerv. Syst.,* 18, 13, 1987.
16. Maggi, C. A., and Meli, A., The sensory-efferent function of capsaicin-sensitive sensory neurons, *Gen. Pharmacol.,* 19, 1, 1988.
17. Holzer, P., Capsaicin: cellular targets, mechanisms of action, and selectivity for thin sensory neurons, *Pharmacol. Rev.,* 43, 143, 1991.
18. Ritter, S., and Dinh, T. T., Capsaicin-induced neuronal degeneration: silver impregnation of cell bodies, axons and terminals in the central nervous system of the adult rat, *J. Comp. Neurol.,* 271, 79, 1988.
19. Ritter, S., and Dinh, T. T., Capsaicin-induced neuronal degeneration in the brain and retina of preweanling rats, *J. Comp. Neurol.,* 296, 447, 1990.
20. McDougal, D. B., Jr., Yuan, M. J. C., Dargar, R. V., and Johnson, E. M., Jr., Neonatal capsaicin and guanethidine and axonally transported organelle-specific enzymes in sciatic nerve and in sympathetic and dorsal root ganglia, *J. Neurosci.,* 3, 124, 1983.
21. Ritter, S., and Taylor, J. S., Capsaicin abolishes lipoprivic but not glucoprivic feeding in rats, *Am. J. Physiol.,* 256, R1232, 1989.
22. Berthoud, H.-R., Carlson, N. R., and Powley, T. L., Topography of efferent vagal innervation of the rat gastrointestinal tract, *Am. J. Physiol.,* 260, R200, 1991.
23. Calingasan, N. Y., and Ritter, S., Presence of galanin in rat vagal sensory neurons: an immunohistochemical and in situ hybridization study, *J. Autonom. Nerv. Syst.,* 40, 229, 1992.
24. Kyrkouli, S. E., Stanley, B. G. and Leibowitz, S. F., Galanin: stimulation of feeding induced by medial hypothalamic injection of this novel peptide, *Eur. J. Pharmacol.,* 122, 159, 1986.
25. Temple, D. L., and Leibowitz, S. F., Diurnal variations in the feeding responses to norepinephrine, neuropeptide Y and galanin in the PVN, *Brain Res. Bull.,* 25, 821, 1990.

26. Leibowitz, S. F., Hypothalamic galanin in relation to feeding behavior and endocrine systems. In: *Galanin: A New Multifunctional Peptide in the Neuroendocrine System,* T. Hokfelt, T. Bartfai, D. Jacobowitz, and D. Ottoson, Eds. Macmillan, New York, 1991, 393.
27. Calingasan, N. Y., Ritter, S., and Kalivas, P. W., Blockade of fatty acid oxidation increases the number of vagal sensory neurons containing galanin mRNA and hnRNA, *Soc. Neurosci. Abstr.,* 18, 896 (#373.7), 1992.
28. Smith, G. P., Jerome, C., Cushin, B. J., Eterno, R., and Simansky, K. J., Abdominal vagotomy blocks the satiety effect of cholecystokinin in the rat, *Science,* 213, 1036, 1981.
29. Ritter, R. C., and Ladenheim, E. E., Capsaicin pretreatment attenuates suppression of food intake by cholecystokinin octapeptide, *Am. J. Physiol.,* 248, R501, 1985.
30. Ritter, S., Calingasan, N. Y., Dinh, T. T., and Taylor, J. S., Expression of c-fos protein is induced in specific brain neurons by metabolic inhibitors that increase food intake, *Neurosci. Abstr.,* 17, 192, 1991.
31. Herbert, H., Moga, M. M., and Saper, C. B., Connections of the parabrachial nucleus with the nucleus of the solitary tract and the medullary reticular formation in the rat, *J. Comp. Neurol.,* 293, 540, 1990.
32. Van der Kooy, D., and Koda, L. Y., Organization of the projections of a circumventricular organ: the area postrema in the rat, *J. Comp. Neurol.,* 219, 328, 1983.
33. Shapiro, R. E., and Miselis, R. R., The central neural connections of the area postrema of the rat, *J. Comp. Neurol.,* 234, 344, 1985.
34. Ricardo, J. A., and Koh, E. T., Anatomical evidence of direct projections from the nucleus of the solitary tract to the hypothalamus, amygdala, and other forebrain structures, *Brain Res.,* 153, 1, 1978.
35. Calingasan, N. Y., and Ritter, S., Lesions of specific lateral parabrachial subnuclei abolish feeding induced by mercaptoacetate but not by 2-deoxy-D-glucose, *Am. J. Physiol.,* in press.
36. Flynn, F. W., Grill, H. J., Schulkin, J., and Norgren, R., Central gustatory lesions. II. Effects on sodium appetitie, taste aversion learning, and feeding behaviors, *Behav. Neurosci.,* 105, 944, 1991.
37. Tordoff, M. G., Geiselman, P. J., Grijalva, C. V., Keifer, S. W., and Novin, D., Amygdaloid lesions impair ingestive responses to 2-deoxy-D-glucose but not insulin, *Am. J. Physiol.,* 242, R129, 1982.
38. Calingasan, N. Y., and Ritter, S., Hypothalamic paraventricular nucleus lesions do not abolish glucoprivic or lipoprivic feeding, *Brain Res.,* in press.
39. Shor-Posner, G., Azar, A., Insinga, S., and Leibowitz, S., Deficits in the control of food intake after hypothalamic paraventricular nucleus lesions, *Physiol. Behav.,* 35, 883, 1985.
40. Morgan, J. I., and Curran, D. R., Calcium and proto-oncogene involvement in the immediate early response in the nervous system, *Ann. N.Y. Acad. Sci.,* 568, 283, 1989.
41. Miselis, R. R., and Epstein, A. N., Feeding induced by intracerebroventricular 2-deoxy-D-glucose in the rat, *Am. J. Physiol.,* 229, 1438, 1975.

42. Ritter, R. C., and Slusser, P. J., 5-Thio-D-glucose causes increased feeding and hyperglycemia in the rat, *Am. J. Physiol.*, 238, E141, 1980.
43. Bird, E., Cardone, C. C., and Contreras, R. J., Area postrema lesions disrupt food intake induced by cerebroventricular infusions of 5-thioglucose in the rat, *Brain Res.*, 270, 193, 1983.
44. Ritter, R. C., Slusser, P. G., and Stone S., Glucoreceptors controlling feeding and blood glucose: location in hindbrain, *Science,* 213, 451, 1981.
45. Contreras, R. J., Fox, E., and Drugovich, M. L., Area postrema lesions produce feeding deficits in the rat: effects of preoperative dieting and 2-deoxy-D-glucose, *Physiol. Behav.*, 29, 875, 1982.
46. Hyde, T. A., and Miselis, R. R., Effects of area postrema/caudal medial nucleus of solitary tract lesions on food intake and body weight, *Am. J. Physiol.*, 244, R577, 1983.
47. Hokfelt, B., and Bydgeman, S., Increased adrenaline production following administration of 2-deoxy-D-glucose in the rat, *Proc. Soc. Exp. Biol. Med.*, 106, 537, 1961.
48. Bellinger, L. L., and Williams, F. E., Aphagia and adipsia after kainic acid lesioning of the dorsomedial hypothalamic area, *Am. J. Physiol.*, 244, R389, 1983.
49. Grossman, S. P., and Grossman, L., Iontophoretic injections of kainic acid into the rat lateral hypothalamus: effects on ingestive behavior, *Physiol. Behav.*, 29, 553, 1982.
50. Bellinger, L. L., and Williams. F. E., Liver denervation does not modify feeding responses to metabolic challenges or hypertonic NaCl induced water consumption, *Physiol. Behav.*, 30, 463, 1983.
51. Tordoff, M. G., Hopfenbeck, J., and Novin, D., Hepatic vagotomy (partial hepatic denervation) does not alter ingestive responses to metabolic challenges, *Physiol. Behav*., 28, 417, 1982.
52. Novin, D., VanderWeele, D. A., and Rezek, M., Infusion of 2-deoxy-D-glucose into the hepatic portal system causes eating: evidence for peripheral glucoreceptors, *Science,* 181, 85, 1973.
53. Russell, P. J. D., and Mogenson, G. J., Drinking and feeding induced by jugular and portal infusions of 2-deoxy-D-glucose, *Am. J. Physiol.*, 229, 1014, 1975.
54. Stricker, E. M., and Rowland, N., Hepatic versus cerebral origin of stimulus for feeding induced by 2-deoxy-D-glucose in rats, *J. Comp. Physiol. Psychol.*, 92, 126, 1978.
55. Delprete, E., and Scharrer, E., Hepatic branch vagotomy attenuates the feeding response to 2-deoxy-d-glucose in rats, *Exp. Physiol.*, 75, 259, 1990.
56. Tordoff, M. G., Rafka, R., DiNovi, M. J., and Friedman, M. I., 2,5-Anhydro-D-mannitol: a fructose analogue that increases food intake in rats, *Am. J. Physiol.*, 254, R150, 1988.
57. Tordoff, M. G., Rawson, N., and Friedman, M. I., 2,5-Anhydro-D-mannitol acts in the liver to initiate feeding, *Am. J. Physiol.*, 261, R283, 1991.
58. Dinh, T. T., Ritter, S., and Friedman, M. I., 2,5-Anhydro-D-mannitol increases Fos-like immunoreactivity (Fos-li) in the AP/NTS region by stimulating vagal sensory neurons, *Soc. Neurosci. Abstr.*, 18, 1067 (#446.10), 1992.

59. Louis-Sylvestre, J., and LeMagnen, J., A fall in blood glucose level precedes meal onset in free-feeding rats, *Neurosci. Biobehav. Rev.*, 4, 13, 1980.
60. Campfield, L. A., Brandon, P., and Smith, F. J., On-line continuous measurement of blood glucose and meal pattern in free-feeding rats: the role of glucose in meal initiation, *Brain Res. Bull.*, 14, 605, 1985.
61. Campfield, L. A., and Smith, F., Systemic factors in the control of food intake. In: *Handbook of Behavioral Neurobiology, Vol. 10: Neurobiology of Food and Fluid Intake,* E. Stricker, Ed. Plenum, New York, 1990, 183.

# *III. Macronutrient Intake, Caloric Compensation, and the Impact of Macronutrient Substitutes*

# Introduction

**Barbara J. Rolls**

Many individuals are worried that they are eating the wrong kinds of foods or that their body weight is too high. There is a widespread concern that intake of dietary fat, and to a lesser extent sugar, should be decreased while intake of fiber should be increased. The food industry has responded to these concerns by producing a wide range of products with reduced fat or sugar contents or with added fiber. This product development often depends on the use of low or zero calorie sugar and fat substitutes that mimic some of the sensory properties of sugar or fat. It is likely that many consumers are choosing foods with reduced sugar or fat, because they expect these foods to have an impact on the composition or energy content of their diet. Readers of the chapters in this section will quickly become aware that it is unwise to make assumptions about how particular constituents of foods will affect food intake or selection.

Food intake can be influenced by many factors including those in the environment, i.e., where and with whom one is eating; those specific to the individual, i.e., age, body weight, previous experience with a food; or those specific to particular foods or drinks, i.e., palatability. The large number of variables involved makes the study of food intake particularly challenging, which is why much of the research examining eating behavior is conducted under rigorous experimental control. Investigators must be cautious, however, about extending their findings beyond a particular experimental paradigm. This is often difficult as the press and the general public are eager for clear messages about how the foods they are eating will affect them. Because of this the results of laboratory-based experiments are sometimes prematurely extrapolated into broad public health messages. To illuminate some of the misconceptions and controversies that have arisen in relation to the effects of diet composition on food intake and body weight, the editors have invited papers from investigators with widely different views. The contributors have done an excellent job of questioning why different studies have yielded different results. At present there are no clear cut answers, but the level of debate indicates that the investigators will continue to examine the critical variables in their studies.

We stand on the brink of what could be some of the biggest changes in diet composition experienced by modern man. The food industry has the capability to eliminate both sugar and fat from a wide variety of foods, and to supplement them with fiber and a range of nutrients. This new food technology will provide investigators studying the regulation of food intake and body weight with exciting new tools for systematically manipulating diet composition. It seems likely that such research will lead to strategies for controlling appetite and food intake.

# 7 Sweetness and Appetite in Normal, Overweight, and Elderly Persons

**Susan S. Schiffman, Zoe S. Warwick, and Maureen Mackey**

## I. INTRODUCTION

Studies of taste in humans have found that there is an innate preference for sweet tastes. However, the degree of liking of strong sweet tastes does vary among individuals. The preference for strong sweet tastes may be due to early childhood experiences or genetic differences in taste or both.

The intensity of sweetness, quality of sweetness, and physiological state affect intake and satiety. Intake of sweet tasting foods is not monotonically related to sweetness intensity. Sweetness is rated as more pleasant during fasting than during nutritional repletion. This chapter will deal more fully with each of these issues, and will discuss sweet taste perception in normal, obese, and elderly persons. The effect of sweet taste on restrained eaters will also be discussed.

## II. HUMAN STUDIES

### A. Innate Preferences for Sweet Taste

Humans are born with the ability to perceive the taste of sugars, as well as other taste qualities.[1] An innate liking for sweet taste has been inferred from the finding that newborns ingest sugar water with more vigor[2] and for a longer time[3] than plain water. Gustofacial responses to the taste of sugar may also reflect a liking for sweet tastes,[4] although these data are difficult to interpret.[5]

### B. Individual Differences

Marked individual differences in hedonic responses to sweet tastes have been reported in adults. "Sweet likers" are persons who perceive the taste

0-8493-4466-2/94/$0.00+$.50

of highly sweet sucrose solutions as pleasant. "Sweet dislikers" are individuals for whom intense sucrose concentrations are perceived as unpleasant. Sweet liker/disliker status is stable during fasted and fed states, although for sweet dislikers, the unpleasantness of strongly sweet solutions is attenuated during fasting.[6] The sweet liker/disliker distinction is also noted when solutions are sweetened with fructose or glucose.[7]

These individual differences in sweet preference may arise from early feeding experiences[8] or from genetic differences in PROP taster status. Sweet likers tend to be nontasters of PROP, while sweet dislikers tend to be PROP tasters.[9] PROP is a compound similar to phenylthiocarbamide (PTC), which has a bimodal threshold distribution.[10] Tasters of PROP are those who detect its bitterness at low concentrations while nontasters require high concentrations to detect the bitter taste. Sweet likers report a more complex gustatory sensation imparted by sucrose solutions, while for sweet dislikers the perceptual experience is more purely sweet.[9]

### C. Sweetness, Appetite, and Food Intake

Two types of studies have been used to evaluate the effect of low-calorie sweeteners on appetite and food intake. The "additive" approach directly tests the effect of perceiving a sweet taste on subsequent responses. In this approach, responses to unsweetened foods are compared to responses to nutritionally identical sweet foods. In the "substitutive" approach, an intense sweetener is substituted for a caloric sweetener in a food, producing a food of equal sweetness but lower caloric content. Since meal sensory properties are equated, this technique is useful for illuminating the effect of nonsensory variables, such as caloric density, on satiety. The substitutive approach is also appropriate for studies of caloric compensation.

In the additive approach, the effect of ingesting a sweetened food/beverage is compared to the effect of ingesting a nutritionally identical, but unsweetened food/beverage on subsequent hunger and food intake. Aspartame, which imparts a clean sweet taste in calorically negligible quantities, frequently has been used to manipulate sweetness without altering the nutritional value of the vehicle. For example, diet soft drinks have been compared with mineral water,[11] and an aspartame sweetened milkshake has been compared with an unsweetened version.[12]

Studies using this approach generally have found no difference in appetite ratings following the sweet and unsweet loads.[11-14] A few studies have found that a sweet meal was actually more satiating, as indicated by a greater decrease in subsequent hunger ratings, than an unsweetened, nutritionally identical meal.[15,16] Mattes concluded, "the present data fail to support a view that sweetness alone stimulates hunger or food intake in a realistic eating situation."[15]

There have been two reports of enhancement of hunger following ingestion of an aqueous aspartame solution[17,18] and one report of increased hunger after chewing aspartame-sweetened gum.[19] In the studies of aqueous aspartame,[17,18] appetite ratings were measured during the hour following ingestion of plain water and were compared to appetite ratings obtained after subjects drank aspartame-sweetened water. It was found that ratings of hunger and of desire to eat were higher following ingestion of the aspartame-sweetened water. In the study using chewing gum, hunger ratings were increased after aspartame-sweetened gum, but the effect was dependent on sex of the subject, concentration of aspartame, and time after chewing.[19]

It is important to note that the studies of aqueous aspartame[17,18] used a relatively high concentration of aspartame: 81 mg/100 ml. This concentration is quite sweet, being equivalent in sweetness intensity to 9.5% sucrose.[20] Although high levels of sweetness are enjoyed when accompanied by flavorings and/or carbonation (for example, in fruit juices or in soda), purely sweet water is typically perceived as less pleasant tasting than plain water.[6] Thus the results of these studies are confounded by the fact that the sweet aqueous solutions may have been unpleasant, or at least were less pleasant than plain water. In a later study from the same laboratory[21] a sweeter solution of aspartame, 117.5 mg/100 ml, resulted in no significant effect on appetite scores compared to plain water. Thus, it is difficult to conclude from these studies whether sweetness stimulates appetite.

Nevertheless, even if one interprets these results as indicating that sweetness stimulates appetite, it is important to recognize that the higher appetite scores observed after consumption of aspartame-sweetened water were not accompanied by increased food intake. In fact, Rogers et al.[18,21] have noted in two separate studies that food intake was marginally lower following consumption of solutions of aspartame. These observations are consistent with the finding of Mattes[22] that there is a poor correlation between hunger ratings and food intake. Numerous other studies have shown that there is no difference in food intake following consumption of aspartame-sweetened or unsweetened beverages.[11-14,23,24] Thus the addition of sweetness to beverages may not affect subsequent food intake.

The results of a study that used saccharin as a sweetening agent for yogurt[25] are inconsistent with those found for aspartame described above. After consuming saccharin-sweetened yogurt, subjects reported feeling less satiated 30 to 60 min later when compared to satiety elicited by equicaloric unsweetened yogurt, and their subsequent food intake was higher following the saccharin-sweetened yogurt compared to the plain yogurt. While Rogers and Blundell[25] attribute this to the sweetness provided by saccharin, this interpretation is not consistent with their observation in the same study that glucose-sweetened yogurt and equicaloric, unsweetened yogurt had similar effects on appetite scores and subsequent food intake.

There has been one study in which the effects of aspartame-sweetened yogurt preloads on subsequent intake were examined.[26] In male subjects there were some differences in 24-h caloric intake following consumption of aspartame-sweetened yogurt preloads of varying sweetness. However, there was no pattern of effect of sweetness intensity on subsequent food intake. In female subjects there were no significant differences in 24-h food intake following consumption of any of the five concentrations of aspartame-sweetened yogurt. Interpretation of this study is made difficult also because no controls were run.

The findings of increased appetite and food intake following consumption of a saccharin-sweetened yogurt[25] also differ from the finding of Mattes[15] who showed consumption of a breakfast including aspartame-sweetened cereal was followed by decreased hunger ratings compared to those for plain or sucrose-sweetened cereals. Energy intakes at lunch and dinner (Figure 3; bottom two panels within Mattes[15]) and over the total day (Table 2 within Mattes[15]) after consumption of aspartame-sweetened vs. plain cereal breakfasts were not significantly different when data for informed and naive subjects were kept appropriately separate. Mattes noted that there was a trend for food intake to be higher among subjects who were informed of the aspartame content of their cereal. However, he concluded that, "...the addition of aspartame or sweet taste to a breakfast cereal had no significant effect on energy intake (at the next meal or over the day), subsequent hunger ratings or selection of items with particular taste characteristics among free-living individuals self-selecting and consuming foods and beverages in their customary diets. Knowledge of sweeteners used exerted a stronger effect on these ingestive behaviors."[15]

In the "substitutive" approach, foods similar in sweetness but differing in caloric content are compared for their effect on subsequent appetite and food intake. Aspartame sweetened foods and beverages, such as gelatin desserts, puddings, and fruit-flavored drinks, have been compared with their sugar-sweetened counterparts. Most studies have shown that consumption of equisweet preloads differing in caloric content results in similar effects on appetite scores.[13,14,27-29] This suggests that appetite is affected more by the volume or bulk of beverage or food, rather than by its caloric content, at least in the short term. Expectations regarding food caloric content also influence appetite and satiety.[30,31] These results do not support those of Blundell and Hill[17] and Rogers et al.[18] who reported that appetite scores were significantly increased following consumption of aspartame-sweetened water whereas those for glucose-sweetened water were suppressed. Measurement of subsequent food intake in these studies showed that there were no significant increases following consumption of the low-calorie preload compared to the high-calorie preload,[13,14,18,29] although in some instances there was a tendency for caloric intake to be slightly higher following the low-calorie preload.[18,27] The data from the study by Rogers and Blundell[25] also indicated that food intakes following the saccharin-sweetened yogurt preloads having 131 cal were not significantly different from those following the glucose-sweetened yogurt having 295 cal.

The results of these studies on short-term caloric compensation following equisweet preloads differing in caloric content suggest that, at least in the short term, caloric compensation is imperfect. It is important to distinguish these studies from long-term studies of caloric compensation[32-34] that used entirely different study protocols, and thus cannot be compared reliably.

Drewnowski et al.[35] recently reported a study that combined the additive and substitutive study designs. They prepared four types of preloads consisting of soft white cheese: A, unsweetened, 300 cal; B, aspartame-sweetened, 300 cal; C, sugar-sweetened, 700 cal; D, aspartame-sweetened, with maltodextrin, 700 cal. Comparison of A vs. B addresses the additive effect, and comparison of B vs. C addresses the substitutive effect. In addition, comparison of C vs. D allows one to assess a unique effect of aspartame on appetite and food intake while both sweetness and calories are controlled. The results showed no effect of sweetness on subsequent intake: food intake following A was similar to that following B. Also, there was no caloric compensation: total daily caloric intake following B was about 400 cal less than that after treatment C, indicating the subjects did not sense the 400 cal difference in preload B and increase subsequent intake to compensate for it. Furthermore, total caloric intake following treatments C and D was similar, adding further support to the conclusion that aspartame does not stimulate subsequent food intake.

Tordoff and Alleva[36] compared the effects of three conditions (aspartame-sweetened soda vs. soda sweetened with high fructose corn sweetener [HFCS] vs. no soda) on food intake and body weight. Caloric and sugar intakes decreased significantly when the subjects consumed aspartame-sweetened soda compared to the no soda and HFCS soda conditions. Also male, but not female subjects lost a significant amount of weight while consuming aspartame-sweetened soda. These findings suggest that use of aspartame-sweetened products when substituted for their sugar-sweetened counterparts can help in creating a caloric deficit that may lead to weight loss. In addition, they also lend further support to the conclusion that aspartame does not stimulate subsequent appetite or food intake.

### D. Effect of Physiological State on Hedonic Response to Sweet Taste

The pleasantness of sweet tastes is related to nutritional state. Sucrose solutions are rated as more pleasant during fasting than following nutritional repletion.[37,38] Studies with rats also show that sweet tastes are more attractive to food-deprived animals.[39-41] Shifts in the pleasantness of sweet tastes as a function of nutritional state, termed "alliesthesia",[42] may play a functional role in food intake regulation. When the body requires calories because internal energy stores have been depleted, sweetness is perceived as highly pleasant, which increases the likelihood of initiating and sustaining a meal. When the gut contains ample energy supplies and therefore calories are not required, sweetness is less attractive, which decreases the likelihood of consumption.

Further evidence of the integration between gustation and nutritional state comes from electrophysiological studies. Neural activity evoked by sugar on the tongue is decreased when internal metabolic conditions mimic a replete state. Exogenous administration of glucose[43] and insulin[44] reduced neural activity elicited by the sweet taste of glucose, but had little effect on responses to the sour taste of hydrochloric acid or the bitter taste of quinine hydrochloride. Nonnutritive stomach distention decreased neural responses to sweet, but not to bitter tastes.[45]

Additional lines of evidence support the hypothesis that changes in the pleasantness of sweetness have functional value. Sweetness is perceived as more pleasant during the luteal phase of the menstrual cycle, and during this time intake of sweet foods increases.[46] Since metabolic rate is elevated during the luteal phase,[47] the heightened palatability and intake of sweet foods during the luteal phase would compensate for increased metabolic energy expenditure. It has also been found that children aged 9 to 15 preferred higher levels of sweetness than did adults.[48] Since adolescents generally have high activity levels and thus high caloric requirements, enhanced preference for sweet tastes may reflect an adaptive response to physiological need.

## E. Response to Sweet Taste in the Elderly

Many elderly persons have markedly impaired olfactory and gustatory acuity.[49-54] Moderate losses occur in the perception of sweet, sour, salty, and bitter tasting compounds as well as amino acids.[54] The losses for smell are more pronounced. The losses for sweet taste occur at both threshold and suprathreshold levels as shown in Tables 1 and 2.[55] The thresholds in Table 1 were determined by a forced choice technique. The age-related losses at threshold are relatively small with an average ratio of threshold (elderly)/threshold (young) of 2.72. The dose-response curves in Table 2 were derived from suprathreshold intensity judgments using the method of magnitude estimation. Young and elderly subjects applied numbers to a range of concentrations of each sweetener so that ratios of the numbers reflected the ratios of the perceived taste intensities. The logs of the concentrations of the sweeteners were plotted against the logs of the

**TABLE 1**
**Mean Detection Thresholds for Sweeteners**

| Stimulus | Young (Y) (m) | Elderly (E) (m) | E/Y |
|---|---|---|---|
| Acesulfam-K | $4.44 \times 10^{-5}$ | $7.47 \times 10^{-5}$ | 1.68 |
| Aspartame | $2.24 \times 10^{-5}$ | $9.13 \times 10^{-5}$ | 4.07 |
| Calcium cyclamate | $2.66 \times 10^{-4}$ | $4.12 \times 10^{-4}$ | 1.55 |
| Fructose | $4.39 \times 10^{-3}$ | $10.1 \times 10^{-3}$ | 2.30 |
| Monellin | $1.95 \times 10^{-8}$ | $9.13 \times 10^{-8}$ | 4.67 |
| Neohesperidin dihydrochalcone | $2.20 \times 10^{-6}$ | $4.60 \times 10^{-6}$ | 2.09 |
| Rebaudioside | $4.61 \times 10^{-6}$ | $13.0 \times 10^{-6}$ | 2.82 |
| Sodium saccharin | $1.47 \times 10^{-5}$ | $4.24 \times 10^{-5}$ | 2.88 |
| Stevioside | $5.31 \times 10^{-6}$ | $16.0 \times 10^{-6}$ | 3.02 |
| Thaumatin | $7.16 \times 10^{-8}$ | $13.3 \times 10^{-8}$ | 1.86 |
| D-Tryptophan | $1.09 \times 10^{-4}$ | $3.22 \times 10^{-4}$ | 2.95 |

From Schiffman et al.[55]

**TABLE 2**
**Slopes of Dose-Response Curves for Sweeteners for Young and Elderly Subjects**

| Stimulus | Young (Y) | Elderly (E) | Loss in elderly (%) |
|---|---|---|---|
| Acesulfam-K | 0.410 | 0.284 | 30.7 |
| Aspartame | 0.454 | 0.284 | 37.4 |
| Calcium cyclamate | 0.548 | 0.366 | 33.2 |
| Fructose | 0.677 | 0.334 | 50.7 |
| Neohesperidin dihydrochalcone | 0.528 | 0.231 | 56.3 |
| Rebaudioside A | 0.704 | 0.300 | 57.4 |
| Sodium saccharin | 0.552 | 0.282 | 48.9 |
| Stevioside | 0.806 | 0.402 | 50.1 |
| Thaumatin | 0.422 | 0.133 | 68.5 |
| D-Tryptophan | 0.905 | 0.417 | 54.0 |

From Schiffman et al.[55]

normalized magnitude estimates yielding straight lines. The slope of the lines that related the log of the concentration (abscissa) to the perceived intensity (ordinate) for each sweetener are given in Table 2. The average decrement in slope is 48.7%. Although these losses in sweet perception do occur with age, preference judgments of sweet-tasting foods suggest that the pleasurable aspects of sweet tastes continue into old age.[49,56,57]

Complaints about the weak flavor of food do occur, however, in the elderly. Although these deficits cannot be reversed, taste and smell losses can be compensated for by increasing the flavor level of foods. Among elderly persons, the pleasantness and intake of food can be enhanced by the addition of intense flavors.[50-54,58]

### F. Taste Preferences in the Obese

Obesity may be partly due to heightened awareness of taste, smell, and textural sensations. Schiffman[59] proposed that a high threshold for sensory satiety contributes to the development and maintenance of obesity. In other words, some individuals require high levels of taste, smell, and texture stimulation to feel satisfied. This preference for high flavor (taste and smell) may promote obesity because high levels of flavor are often found in high-fat foods. Foods that are high in fat (and caloric density) are highly reinforcing. Support for this hypothesis of heightened sensory satiety threshold emerged from a study in which obese persons were placed on a low-calorie diet that incorporated high levels of noncaloric flavors. On this regimen, overweight persons felt satisfied and thus were able to maintain the diet and achieve weight loss.[59]

More recently, it was found that supplementing a low-calorie diet with aspartame improved dietary adherence.[60] Obese women were placed on a hypocaloric diet for 12 weeks: half of the women were advised to include aspartame-sweetened products in the diet, while the remaining women were instructed to avoid aspartame-containing food. The main finding was that obese women assigned to a diet including aspartame-sweetened foods lost as much weight as women following a nutritionally identical diet without aspartame-sweetened foods. The association between aspartame usage and greater weight loss was evidence for closer compliance with the hypocaloric dietary guidelines. In other words, women consuming a diet with free access to low calorie or calorie-free sweet foods and beverages were better able to stick to the diet. A 1-year follow-up study of long-term weight maintenance has shown that users of aspartame-sweetened products are significantly more likely than nonusers to avoid regaining the weight they had lost.[61]

Sweetness has also been associated with increased metabolic rate.[62] Human subjects who tasted a sweet food, but did not swallow it, had increased energy expenditure that was not attributable to oromotor activity.

### G. Taste Preferences in Restrained Eaters

Persons who are chronically dieting and are preoccupied with food and body weight are termed "restrained eaters".[63] Restrained eaters typically consume fewer calories per day than unrestrained eaters.[64] However, this caloric restriction is punctuated by episodes of ingesting large quantities of calories. Sweet foods are more likely to be the target of binge eating than are nonsweet foods.[65,66] The attractiveness of sweet foods may stem from their potential to rectify a deficit in orosensory stimulation.

Orosensory stimulation is an important component of satiety,[67-71] in that a meal is less satiating when it is unaccompanied by orosensory stimulation. It is noteworthy that dieters typically consume foods perceived as "diet-friendly", such as cottage cheese, salad, plain poultry, and fruit. These foods are not very satiating from a sensory standpoint since they provide little taste and smell stimulation, and have bland textures. Therefore, chronic dieters incur a deficit in orosensory stimulation, in addition to the intended deficit in calories. This reasoning suggests that sweet foods may be highly attractive to restrained eaters due to their potent sensory impact and palatability, which acts to ameliorate the self-imposed deficit in orosensory satiety.

## III. ANIMAL STUDIES

### A. Innate Preference for Sweet Taste

An innate preference for the taste of sugars is also noted in rats. Neonatal rats exhibit positive ingestive responses to oral infusions of sucrose solutions[72,73] and complex carbohydrates.[74] Sodium saccharin also elicits positive ingestive responses in 12-day-old rats.[75,76]

### B. Sweetness, Appetite, and Food Intake

In rats, saccharin stimulates short-term consumption, but typically does not increase long-term calorie intake. During short-term preference tests, rats ate more saccharin-sweetened than unsweetened diet.[77] Over a period of weeks, saccharin stimulated intake and weight gain when it was mixed into a wet diet containing 80% water but not with a wet diet containing 60% water. Saccharin did not affect intake when consumed as a separate solution. The saccharin-induced stimulation of intake was obliterated when the rats were previously exposed for several days to an unsweetened plain diet or to saccharin in water prior to introduction of the sweetened diets.[77] *Ad libitum* cyclamate solution did not affect food intake by mice during a 23-day period.[78]

### C. Sweetness and Satiety

In rats, sweet taste enhances the satiating effect of systemically injected nutrient. Animals ate less when given an intraportal load of glucose in conjunction with a sweet taste than when given the intraportal glucose with no taste stimulation.[79] In a similar manner, intraperitoneal glucose paired with a taste suppressed sham-feeding to a greater extent than intraperitoneal glucose in the absence of taste.[71] These findings are consistent with other studies in rats that illustrate that satiety is enhanced by oral stimulation.[67,80,81]

## IV. SUMMARY

Preference for sweet taste is innate in humans and animals. There are marked individual differences in adults, however, which may be due to early feeding experiences and genetic differences in the ability to taste 6-*n*-propylthiouracil. Physiological state can also modify sweet taste preferences. The preference for sweet taste lasts into old age.

Numerous studies have shown that sweetness does not stimulate subsequent appetite and food intake. The use of intense sweeteners instead of sugar in foods can create a caloric deficit that may not elicit caloric compensation. Dieters who use aspartame-sweetened products may be more successful at weight loss and long-term weight maintenance. This success may be related to the amount of aspartame-sweetened products used, and to the conscious effort by dieters to use the products to help them create a caloric deficit.

## ACKNOWLEDGMENT

Supported by NIA Grant AGO0443 to S. S. Schiffman.

## REFERENCES

1. Lipsitt, L. P., and Behl, G., Taste-mediated differences in the sucking behavior of human newborns. In: *Taste, Experience, and Feeding,* E. D. Capaldi, and T. L. Powley, Eds., American Psychological Association, Washington D.C., 1990, 75.
2. Nowlis, G. H., and Kessen, W., Human newborns differentiate differing concentrations of sucrose and glucose, *Science,* 191, 865, 1976.
3. Crook, C. K., Taste perception in the newborn infant, *Infant Behav. Dev.,* 1, 52,1978.
4. Steiner, J. E., The human gustofacial response. In: *Fourth Symposium on Oral Sensation and Perception. Development in the Fetus and Infant,* J. F. Bosma, Ed., National Institutes of Health [DHEW publication No. (NIH) 73-546], Bethesda, MD, 1973, 254.
5. Cowart, B. J., and Beauchamp, G. K., Early development of taste perception. In: *Psychological Basis of Sensory Evaluation,* R. McBride and H. MacFie, Eds., Elsevier, Barking, England, 1990.

6. Looy, H., and Weingarten, H. P., Effects of metabolic state on sweet taste reactivity in humans depend on underlying response profile, *Chem. Senses,* 16, 123,1991.
7. Looy, H., Callaghan, S., and Weingarten, H. P., Hedonic response of sucrose likers and dislikers to other gustatory stimuli, *Physiol. Behav.,* 52, 219, 1992.
8. Beauchamp, G. K., and Moran, M., Dietary experience and sweet taste preference in human infants, *Appetite,* 3, 139,1982.
9. Looy, H., and Weingarten, H. P., Facial expressions and genetic sensitivity to 6-*n*-propylthiouracil predict hedonic response to sweet, *Physiol. Behav.,* 52, 75, 1992.
10. Whissell-Buechy, D., Genetic basis of the phenylthiocarbamide polymorphism, *Chem. Senses,* 15, 27,1990.
11. Black, R. M., Tanaka, P. A., Leiter, L. A., and Anderson, G. H., Soft drinks with aspartame: effect on subjective hunger, food selection, and food intake of young adult males, *Physiol. Behav.,* 49, 803,1991.
12. Brala, P. M., and Hagen, R. L., Effects of sweetness perception and caloric value of a preload on short term intake, *Physiol. Behav.,* 30, 1, 1983.
13. Canty, P. J., and Chan, M. M., Effects of consumption of caloric vs. noncaloric sweet drinks on indices of hunger and food consumption in normal adults, *Am. J. Clin. Nutr.,* 53, 1159, 1991.
14. Rolls, B. J., Kim, S., and Federoff, I. C., Effects of drinks sweetened with sucrose or aspartame on hunger, thirst and food intake in men, *Physiol. Behav.,* 48, 19, 1990.
15. Mattes, R., Effects of aspartame and sucrose in hunger and energy intake in humans, *Physiol. Behav.,* 47, 1037, 1990.
16. Warwick, Z. S., and Schiffman, S. S., Effect of meal sensory properties on postprandial hunger and taste reactivity in human subjects. Fourteenth Annual Meeting of the Association of Chemoreception Science, Sarasota, 1992.
17. Blundell, J. E., and Hill, A. J., Paradoxical effects of an intense sweetener (aspartame) on appetite, *Lancet,* i, 1092, 1986.
18. Rogers, P. J., Carlyle, J., Hill, A. J., and Blundell, J. E., Uncoupling sweet taste and calories: comparison of the effects of glucose and three intense sweeteners on hunger and food intake, *Physiol. Behav.,* 43, 547, 1988.
19. Tordoff, M. G., and Alleva, A. M., Oral stimulation with aspartame increases hunger, *Physiol. Behav.,* 47, 555, 1990.
20. DuBois, G. E., Walters, D. E., Schiffman, S. S., Warwick, Z. S., Booth, B. J., Pecore, S. J., Gibes, K., Carr, B. T., and Brands, L. M., Concentration-response relationships among sweeteners: a systematic study. In: *Sweeteners: Discovery, Molecular Design, and Chemoreception,* F. T. Orthoefer, and G. E. DuBois, Eds. American Chemical Society Symposium Ser. No. 450, Washington D.C., 1990.
21. Rogers, P. J., Pleming, H. C., and Blundell J. E., Aspartame ingested without tasting inhibits hunger and food intake, *Physiol. Behav.,* 47, 1239, 1990.
22. Mattes, R., Hunger ratings are not a valid proxy measure of reported food intake in humans, *Appetite,* 15, 103, 1990.
23. Rodin, J., Comparative effects of fructose, aspartame, glucose, and water preloads on calorie and macronutrient intake, *Am. J. Clin. Nutr.,* 51, 428, 1990.

24. Birch, L. L., McPhee, L., and Sullivan, S., Children's food intake following drinks sweetened with sucrose or aspartame: time course effects, *Physiol. Behav.,* 45, 387, 1989.
25. Rogers, P. J., and Blundell, J. E., Separating the actions of sweetness and calories: effects of saccharin and carbohydrates on hunger and food intake in human subjects, *Physiol. Behav.,* 45, 1093, 1989.
26. Monneuse, M. O., Bellisle, F., and Louis-Sylvestre, J. L., Responses to an intense sweetener in humans: immediate preference and delayed effects on intake, *Physiol. Behav.,* 49, 325, 1991.
27. Rolls, B. J., Hetherington, M., and Laster, L. J., Comparison of the effects of aspartame and sucrose on appetite and food intake, *Appetite,* 11 (Suppl.), 62, 1988.
28. Rolls, B. J., Laster, L. J., and Summerfelt, A., Hunger and food intake following consumption of low-calorie foods, *Appetite,* 13, 115, 1989.
29. Anderson, G. H., Saravis, S., Schacher, R., Zlotkin, S., and Leiter, L. A., Aspartame: effect on lunchtime food intake, appetite and hedonic response in children, *Appetite,* 13, 93, 1989.
30. Booth, D. A., Lee, M., and McAleavey, C., Acquired sensory control of satiation in man, *Br. J. Psychol.,* 67, 137, 1976.
31. Tepper, B. J., Mattes, R. D., and Farkas, B. K., Learned flavor cues influence food intake in humans, *J. Sensory Stud.,* 6, 89, 1991.
32. Foltin, R. W., Fischman, M. W., Moran, T. H., Rolls, B. J., and Kelly, T. H., Caloric compensation for lunches varying in fat and carbohydrate content by humans in a residential laboratory, *Am. J. Clin. Nutr.,* 52, 969, 1990.
33. Foltin, R. W., Rolls, B. J., Moran, T. H., Kelly, T. H., McNelis, A. L., and Fischman, M. W., Caloric, but not macronutrient, compensation by humans for required-eating occasions with meals and snack varying in fat and carbohydrate, *Am. J. Clin. Nutr.,* 55, 331, 1992.
34. Caputo, F. A., and Mattes, R. D., Human dietary responses to covert manipulations of energy, fat, and carbohydrate in a midday meal, *Am. J. Clin. Nutr.,* 56, 36, 1992.
35. Drewnowski, A., Louis-Sylvestre, J., Massein, C., Fricker, J., Chapelot, D., and Apfelbaum, M., Effects of sucrose and aspartame on hunger, energy intake and taste responsiveness in normal-weight men and women. Abstract presented at the Annual Meeting, Society for the Study of Ingestive Behavior, Princeton, NJ, June 1992.
36. Tordoff, M. G., and Alleva, A. M., Effect of drinking soda sweetened with aspartame or high-fructose corn syrup on food intake and body weight, *Am. J. Clin. Nutr.,* 51, 963, 1990.
37. Cabanac, M., and Duclaux, R., Specificity of internal signals in producing satiety for taste stimuli, *Nature (London),* 227, 966, 1970.
38. Fantino, M., Hosotte, J., and Apfelbaum, M., An opioid antagonist, naltrexone, reduces preference for sucrose in humans, *Am. J. Physiol.,* 251, R91, 1986.
39. Cabanac, M., and Lafrance, L., Postingestive alliesthesia: the rat tells the same story, *Physiol. Behav.,* 47, 539, 1990.
40. Cabanac, M., and Lafrance, L., Ingestive/aversive response of rats to sweet stimuli. Influences of glucose, oil, and casein hydrolyzate gastric loads, *Physiol. Behav.,* 51, 139, 1992.

41. Berridge, K. C., Modulation of taste affect by hunger, caloric satiety, and sensory-specific satiety in the rat, *Appetite,* 16, 103, 1991.
42. Cabanac, M., Physiological role of pleasure, *Science,* 173, 1103, 1971.
43. Giza, B. K., and Scott, T. R., Blood glucose selectively affects taste-evoked activity in rat nucleus tractus solitarius, *Physiol. Behav.,* 31, 643, 1983.
44. Giza, B. K., and Scott, T. R., Intravenous insulin infusions decrease gustatory-evoked responses to sugars, *Am. J. Physiol.,* 252, R994, 1987.
45. Glenn, J. F., and Erickson, R. P., Gastric modulation of gustatory afferent activity, *Physiol. Behav.,* 16, 561, 1976.
46. Bowen, D. J., and Grunberg, N. E., Variations in food preference and consumption across the menstrual cycle, *Physiol. Behav.,* 47, 287, 1990.
47. Webb, P., Energy expenditure and the menstrual cycle, *Am. J. Clin. Nutr.,* 44, 614, 1986.
48. Desor, J., Greene, L., and Maller, O., Preferences for sweet and salty in 9- to 15-year old humans, *Science,* 190, 686, 1975.
49. Schiffman, S., Food recognition by the elderly, *J. Gerontol.,* 32, 586, 1977.
50. Schiffman, S., Changes in taste and smell with age: psychophysical aspects. In: *Sensory Systems and Communication in the Elderly,* (Aging, Vol. 10), J. M. Ordy and K. Brizzee, Eds. Raven Press, New York, 1979, 227.
51. Schiffman, S. S., Taste and smell in disease, *N. Engl. J. Med.,* 308, 1275; 1337; 1983.
52. Schiffman, S. S., Smell. In: *Encyclopedia of Aging,* G. L. Maddox, Ed. Springer, New York, 1987, 618.
53. Schiffman, S. S., Taste. In: *Encyclopedia of Aging,* G. L. Maddox, Ed. Springer, New York, 1987, 655.
54. Schiffman, S. S., Taste and smell perception in elderly persons. In: *Nutrition Research: Future Directions and Applications,* J. E. Fielding, and H. I. Frier, Eds. Raven Press, New York, 1991, 61.
55. Schiffman, S. S., Lindley, M. G., Clark, T. B., and Makino, C., Molecular mechanism of sweet taste: relationship of hydrogen bonding to taste sensitivity for both young and elderly, *Neurobiol. Aging,* 2, 173, 1981.
56. Schiffman, S. S., and Covey, E., Changes in taste and smell with age: nutritional aspects. In: *Nutrition in Gerontology,* J. M. Ordy, D. Harman, and R. Alfin-Slater, Eds. Raven Press, New York, 1984, 43.
57. Warwick, Z. S., and Schiffman, S. S., Sensory evaluations of fat-sucrose and fat-salt mixtures: relationship to age and weight status, *Physiol. Behav.,* 48, 633, 1990.
58. Schiffman, S. S., and Warwick, Z. S., Flavor enhancement of foods for the elderly can reverse anorexia, *Neurobiol. Aging,* 9, 24, 1988.
59. Schiffman, S. S., The use of flavor to enhance efficacy of reducing diets, *Hosp. Pract.,* July, 44H, 1986.
60. Kanders, B. S., Lavin, P. T., Kowalchuk, M. B., Greenberg, I., and Blackburn, G. L., An evaluation of the effect of aspartame on weight loss, *Appetite,* 11 (Suppl.), 73, 1988.
61. Kanders, B., Blackburn, G., Lavin, P., Whatley, J., Keller, S., and Conaway, B., Aspartame facilitates longterm weight maintenance in a population of reduced obese women undergoing multidisciplinary treatment for obesity. Meeting of the North American Association for the Study of Obesity/Society for the Study of Ingestive Behavior, Sacramento, CA, 1991.

62. LeBlanc, J., and Cabanac, M., Cephalic postprandial thermogenesis in human subjects, *Physiol. Behav.,* 46, 479, 1989.
63. Herman, C. P., and Mack, D., Restrained and unrestrained eating, *J. Person.,* 43, 647, 1975.
64. Laessle, R. G., Tuschl, R. J., Kotthaus, B. C., and Pirke, K. M., Behavioral and biological correlates of dietary restraint in normal life, *Appetite,* 12, 83, 1989.
65. Tomarken, A. J., and Kirschenbaum, D. S., Effects of plans for future meals on counterregulatory eating by restrained and unrestrained eaters, *J. Ab. Psychol.,* 93, 458, 1984.
66. Warwick, Z. S., Costanzo, P. R., and Schiffman, S. S., Differential response to sweetness, saltiness, and taste variety by restrained vs. unrestrained eaters, *Proc. Ann. Meeting Eastern Psychol. Assoc.,* Philadelphia, PA, 34, 1990.
67. Antin, J., Gibbs, J., and Smith, G. P., Intestinal satiety requires pregastric food stimulation, *Physiol. Behav.,* 18, 421, 1977.
68. Jordan, H. A., Voluntary intragastric feeding: oral and gastric contributions to food intake and hunger in man, *J. Comp. Physiol. Psychol.,* 68, 498, 1969.
69. Wolf, S., and Wolff, H. G., *Human Gastric Function,* Oxford University Press, London, 1947.
70. Taylor, R., Hunger in the infant, *Am. J. Dis. Child.,* 14, 233, 1917.
71. Bedard, M., and Weingarten, H. P., Postabsorptive glucose decreases excitatory effects of taste on ingestion, *Am. J. Physiol.,* 256, R1142, 1989.
72. Hall, W. G., and Bryan T. E., The ontogeny of feeding in rats. IV. Taste development as measured by intake and behavioral responses to oral infusions of sucrose and quinine, *J. Comp. Physiol. Psychol.,* 95, 240, 1981.
73. Ackroff, K., Vigorito, M., and Sclafani, A., Fat appetite in rats: the response of infant and adult rats to nutritive and non-nutritive oil emulsions, *Appetite,* 15, 171, 1990.
74. Vigorito, M., and Sclafani, A., Ontogeny of polycose and sucrose appetite in neonatal rats, *Dev. Psychobiol.,* 21, 457, 1988.
75. Jacobs, H. L., Observations on the ontogeny of saccharine preference in the neonate rat, *Psychon. Sci.,* 1, 105, 1964.
76. Swithers-Mulvey, S. E., and Hall, W. G., Control of ingestion by oral habituation in rat pups, *Behav. Neurosci.,* 106(4), 710–717, 1992.
77. Ramirez, I., Stimulation of energy intake and growth by saccharin in rats, *J. Nutr.,* 120, 123, 1990.
78. Friedhoff, R., Simon, J. A., and Friedhoff, A. J., Sucrose solution vs. no-calorie sweetener vs. water in weight gain, *J. Am. Diet. Assoc.,* 59, 485, 1971.
79. Novin, D., Robinson, K., Culbreth, L. A., and Tordoff, M. G., Is there a role for the liver in the control of food intake?, *Am. J. Clin. Nutr.,* 42, 1050, 1985.
80. Kohn, M., Satiation of hunger from food injected directly into the stomach versus food ingested by mouth, *J. Comp. Physiol. Psychol.,* 44, 412, 1951.
81. Berkun, M. M., Kessen, M. L., and Miller, N. E., Hunger-reducing effects of food by stomach fistula versus food by mouth measured by a consummatory response, *J. Comp. Physiol. Psychol.,* 45, 550, 1952.

# 8 Sweet Carbohydrate Substitutes (Intense Sweeteners) and the Control of Appetite: Scientific Issues

**John E. Blundell and Peter J. Rogers**

## I. APPETITE — RESTRAINED BY SWEETNESS, CARBOHYDRATES, OR BOTH?

For several years intense sweeteners have been welcomed as a means to reduce energy intake, and it has sometimes been claimed that they can be used as dietary aids to produce weight loss. This implies that intense sweeteners can restrain the expression of human appetite. In practice, intense sweeteners replace sweet carbohydrates in dietary products. Does this replacement (which creates a caloric deficit) lead to caloric compensation; and what are the biological actions and appetite effects of the intense sweeteners when given alone?

An understanding of the role of sweeteners in the control of appetite has important theoretical and practical implications. Sweetness is a particularly potent psychobiological phenomenon. Humans show a strong preference for sweet tasting stimuli that appears to have an innate basis, and human beings of all ages find sweet foods and beverages highly acceptable. Indeed, it is likely that sweetness is an important dimension influencing food choice, having a positive promoting effect on human appetite. Consequently, investigations of the mechanisms that mediate the effects of sweetness can help to throw light on the scientific basis of the expression of appetite. Furthermore, it follows that sweetness could have important practical implications in matters concerning human food consumption. This includes the role of

0-8493-4466-2/94/$0.00+$.50

sweetness of foods in those cultures in which there is an abundance of food and where obesity is a major health hazard.

## II. RECENT VIEWS ON THE EFFECTS OF SWEETNESS ON APPETITE AND SATIETY

Since sweetness is often associated with the presence of energy in carbohydrate-rich foods, an examination of the role of sweet foods must embrace a consideration of the separate contributions made by sweetness per se and by calories. Intense sweeteners assume particular importance because they provide a high level of sweetness without (or with very few) calories. One recurrent issue concerns the capacity of intense sweeteners to bring about satiety and therefore to produce effective control of appetite. A recent review[1] has provided a selective appreciation of some experiments on this issue. We believe that this review did not do justice to the complexity of the mechanisms involved and presented an incomplete picture of the possible actions of intense sweeteners. The present chapter outlines a psychobiological view that attempts to resolve some of the scientific issues involved in this field. In turn, this provides a basis for evaluating the practical contributions that intense sweeteners can make in the control of human appetite.

In the opinion of a previous reviewer[1] all acceptable studies on the satiating power of intense sweeteners demonstrate an adequate control of energy intake; some studies that indicate the opposite are either omitted or the results are not fully reported. For example, the thorough study of Brala and Hagen[2] that reported aspartame-induced increases in intake (9% more than placebo control, 26% more than sucrose) is not even mentioned. In a more recent study, Mattes[3] compared the effects of equicaloric breakfasts sweetened with aspartame or sucrose with an unsweetened breakfast. Analysis of subsequent food intake (lunch, dinner, snacks) revealed a significant cereal × meal interaction. "Post hoc tests indicated that lunch and dinner meals were significantly larger following the aspartame cereal than after either the plain or sucrose-sweetened cereal" (Mattes,[3] p. 1040). This effect can be seen clearly in the top panel of Figure 3 (Mattes,[3] p. 1041).* In the review of the effects of these breakfast cereals in the Mattes study, it is

* The highest intakes at both lunch and dinner were observed in subjects who were informed that they were consuming an aspartame-sweetened cereal. While "naive" subjects (not told about the type of sweetener used) also tended to consume more following aspartame, the effect was smaller, although not significantly so, than for the informed subjects. One possibility, therefore, is that the significantly larger intakes were due to some direct effect of aspartame. However, the interpretation favored by Mattes is that subjects informed about the presence of aspartame consciously compensated (or perhaps relaxed

commented that "there were no significant differences in intake of the next meal ..." (Rolls,[1] p. 875). This is only a partial reflection of the outcome of the experiment. Scientists who follow this field of research closely will be able to make an informed evaluation of these comments. However, the casual reader, without the benefit of this more detailed knowledge of the field, will be left with quite a different picture.

There is also a significant change in the interpretation of studies emanating from the work of one group that is accompanied by a change in the actual experimental outcomes. For example, the early studies indicated that "... high intensity sweeteners such as aspartame in foods did not differ substantially from sucrose in how they influenced . . . subsequent food intake" (Rolls et al.,[4] p. 66). In other words, "adults who were offered jello sweetened with either sucrose or aspartame . . . despite the difference in calories consumed . . . [showed] no compensation for the caloric difference an hour later" (Rolls,[5] p. 169). In contrast, in a later study, the carbohydrate content of lunch was reduced and "most of the manipulation was due to the substitution of aspartame for sugar. They [the subjects] made up for the difference in calories in the lunches every day of the experiment and this compensation was seen by dinner time" (Rolls,[1] p. 876 describing the study by Foltin et al.[6]). These findings are reported as if they pose no problem. However, this later study demonstrates compensation while the earlier studies apparently fail to do so. This inconsistency should be explained, for the later study[6] suggests that substituted carbohydrates do not offer any special advantage to the consumer for controlling appetite, whereas the earlier studies all indicated an optimistic view of calorie saving based on the concept of a component of satiety mediated by sensory contact with food.

An examination of the methodology of the so-called sensory-specific satiety experiments[7] indicates that a great deal of interference with sensations, cognitions, behavior, and metabolism occurred in the interval between the consumption of the manipulated products (the preload) and the test of energy adjustment. Usually at 2, 20, 40, and 60 min after the consumption of products subjects were, on each occasion, offered nine samples (each weighing up to 5 g) of foods to taste and rate. Subjects were instructed to swallow the sample after each rating. As far as we are aware no details have been reported on the total energy or nutrient content of the foods swallowed during the interval between preload and test meal. Nor has any account been taken of the interference with afferent processing due to the iterative stimulation of

* (Continued). their eating restraint) for what they assumed, incorrectly, to be a reduced-energy breakfast. Since under normal eating conditions consumers are generally aware of whether a product contains a low-energy sweetener substitute or not, such a response could well help to undermine self-imposed dietary control (see also Conclusions below). Indeed, in discussing this issue Mattes[3] concludes that "the present data raise questions regarding the potential efficacy of aspartame as an aid in weight management regimens" (p. 1043).

olfactory, oral, and gastrointestinal receptors. However, it is difficult to believe that this experimental contamination (amounting to the sampling of 36 food items and swallowing up to 180 g of food) would not compromise the validity of the test meal as indicator of the energy value of the preload. Consequently, it may be considered that many experiments that appeared to give credibility to a strong influence of sensory satiety overriding caloric compensation were methodologically flawed.

It is our view that an earlier review[1] of this field fails to address adequately the complexity of the scientific issues underlying the effects of intense sweeteners and substituted carbohydrates on appetite control. A good deal of the apparent confusion can be elucidated by considering two major issues. One issue concerns the additive and substitutive strategies, and the other involves the postingestive actions of intense sweeteners.

## III. ADDITIVE AND SUBSTITUTIVE PRINCIPLES

This first issue seeks to elucidate the effect of sweetness per se separate from the action of calories that may or may not accompany the sweetness. We have demonstrated on many occasions that sweetness per se can stimulate hunger and/or food intake, while calories have the opposite effect (usually reducing hunger and intake).[8-14] This is illustrated by some recent data[11] shown in Table 1. Food intake at lunch was reduced 1 h following the consumption of a glucose-sweetened yogurt compared with that after eating an equally sweet aspartame-sweetened yogurt, resulting in very similar overall intakes (preload plus lunch). However, overall intakes were higher when the sweet yogurts (glucose or aspartame) were eaten than when an unsweetened yogurt was given as the preload. Particularly important is the finding that lunch intake was significantly greater after the aspartame-sweetened yogurt compared with the unsweetened yogurt, since these preloads differ only in sweetness. Preference (palatability) is not a confounding factor because subjects were recruited on the basis that they liked to eat both sweetened and unsweetened yogurt. Also in this study the subjects were not informed of the type of sweetener used, nor were they told about the differing energy content of the yogurts.

The demonstration of the separate actions of sweetness and calories requires the use of strong experimental designs that allow the uncoupling or disengagement of these two factors.[15] The additive principle applies when, for example, an intense sweetener is added to an unsweetened food. Then a comparison can be made between the effects of two isocaloric products that differ in sweetness. In this way the effects of sweetness can be assessed while holding energy constant. The substitutive principle applies when two products

**TABLE 1**
**Effects of Feeding Sweetened and Unsweetened Yogurt Preloads on Subsequent Test Meal Intake**

| | Mean ± SE energy intakes (kcal) | |
|---|---|---|
| | **Preload** | **Lunch** |
| Unsweetened preload | 131 | 821 ± 54 |
| Aspartame-sweetened preload | 131 | 887 ± 61[a] |
| Glucose-sweetened preload | 295 | 744 ± 52 |

[a] Significantly different from unsweetened and glucose ($p < 0.05$; repeated measures design, $n = 23$). Add fixed preload to lunch intake to get overall intake (see text for further discussion).

are compared that are equivalent in sweetness but differ in energy value. In this way the action of calories can be compared while holding sweetness constant. The strongest experimental designs involve experiments that contain tests of both the additive and the substitutive principles (see Rogers and Blundell[16] for review). It is important to note that the effect of sweetness per se can be evaluated only in those studies that incorporate the additive principle, and it is on the basis of these studies that a stimulating effect of sweetness can be detected. It follows that experiments which incorporate only the substitutive principle[4,7] cannot possibly disclose effects of sweetness per se, since sweetness has not been manipulated as an independent variable (it has been kept constant).

Examination of the effects of the substitutive principle in our studies, with preservation of the cleanliness of the interval between preload and test meal, have always demonstrated that effects of differences in the carbohydrate (energy) content of the preload can be detected 1 h later. These studies have demonstrated the satiating capacity of various carbohydrates (glucose, sucrose, fructose, and starches), and therefore constitute evidence for a short-term energo-static control of appetite (see Rogers and Blundell[16] for review). In contrast, some other studies that involve the substitutive principle have failed to demonstrate consistent and reliable differences in test meal intakes following manipulated preloads.[4] In other words, a satiating effect of carbohydrates was not observed. As pointed out earlier, the interpretation of these data is hindered by the contamination of psychobiological processes during the preload–test meal interval.

Whatever interpretation is placed on the caloric compensation aspects of the sensory-specific satiety studies, investigators should keep in mind the essential differences that can (and cannot) be disclosed by the additive and substitutive principles. A consideration of these principles makes it clear that the satiating capacity of a sweet food will be determined by its energy value and sweetness acting conjointly. A number of studies have indicated that calories per se suppress later intake while sweetness tends to oppose this effect (see Table 1).[10-12] For instance, glucose is less satiating than an equicaloric amount of starch, and aspartame-sweetened food is less satiating than the same food left unsweetened (additive principle). Furthermore, saccharin- or aspartame-sweetened food is less satiating than the same food sweetened with glucose (substitutive principle). Consequently, it can be deduced that sweetness tends to weaken the satiating power of the caloric content of food. In our studies using the additive principle we have referred to the difference in test meal intakes (following sweet or nonsweet equicaloric preloads) as reflecting a stimulatory effect of sweetness on later consumption. However, it is probably more appropriate biologically to refer to this effect as an action of sweetness weakening satiety.

In this context it is also worth pointing out that we have never claimed that aspartame per se can stimulate appetite. Only that sweetness (mediated by aspartame, saccharin, sucrose, etc.) per se will stimulate appetite when the additive principle is operative. To the best of our knowledge, the only study that has demonstrated a stimulatory effect of aspartame (over and above sweetness — that is when isosweet conditions exist) is the report by Mattes.[3]

One further aspect of the substitution of sweet carbohydrates by caloric sweeteners concerns the demand for carbohydrate by the body. There is now good evidence that because stores of carbohydrate in the body are small and this is the preferred fuel for oxidation, there is a high turnover of carbohydrates coupled with a strong impulse for carbohydrate intake.[17,18] Substituting for carbohydrate will compromise this mechanism and may stimulate compensatory seeking for energy in high-fat foods. Some evidence of such an effect can be seen in studies involving large scale substitution of aspartame in foods.[19] Given the apparent importance of this mechanism as a factor in body weight control,[20] this aspect of carbohydrate substitution should be examined more closely.[21]

## IV. POSTINGESTIVE ACTIONS OF INTENSE SWEETENERS

A further important aspect of the effects of intense sweeteners revealed by recent research concerns their actions on postingestive mechanisms.

In a study in which we fed subjects yogurt preloads sweetened with saccharin or glucose or supplemented with starch we observed increases in subsequent food intake due to the effects of sweetness and further longer term increases in intake specific to saccharin.[10] Contrary to the suggestion of Rolls[1] (p. 873), these results cannot be explained by palatability differences, since only volunteers who liked both sweetened and unsweetened yogurts were selected for the study. As in the study summarized in Table 1, great care was taken to ensure that preference was not a confounding factor, and this was confirmed by hedonic ratings of the yogurt preloads (Table 3, in Rogers and Blundell[10]). These findings suggest that saccharin can influence appetite due to its sweet taste and also due to effects on postingestive mechanisms. Consistent with this conclusion, previous work has identified a number of physiological actions of saccharin that could mediate increases in food intake.[10,14]

In addition to these results with saccharin we have also found that aspartame can influence appetite via a postingestive effect — aspartame administered in capsules *reduced* food intake in a test meal eaten 1 h later.[22,23] Thus different intense sweeteners can have different effects on appetite, a conclusion that also applies to sugars.[24] It is important to note that the inhibition of food intake by capsulated aspartame is a robust finding, notwithstanding the report of a negative result in an earlier study[25] from which it was concluded that neither phenylalanine nor aspartame reduces food intake in humans. In that study, alanine was used as the "placebo" treatment, and a careful examination of the data suggests that this was an inappropriate control. Data for four doses of phenylalanine (0.84–10.08 g) are reported. These show a dose-dependent decrease in food intake from 1543 to 1070 kcal. Food intakes after the highest doses (10.08 g) of alanine and aspartame were 1230 and 1124 kcal, respectively. We have reanalyzed these data (available from the Ph.D. thesis[26] on which the published paper[25] was based) and the results are plotted in Figure 1. Taken together with our findings these data suggest that aspartame, phenylalanine, and perhaps alanine all suppress food intake. Aspartame, however, is by far the most potent treatment, for example, 235 mg aspartame (equivalent to the amount of aspartame contained in one to two cans of certain "diet" sodas) reduced test meal intake by between 9 and 14% (138 and 175 kcal).[22,23] The similar suppression of intake by the highest doses of aspartame and phenylalanine in the experiments of Ryan-Harshman et al.[25] may indicate the maximal or asymptotic effect of aspartame, at least under these conditions. Therefore, there is strong evidence that when administered in capsules these substances are anorexic, with the dose-response curve for aspartame to the left of that for phenylalanine.[27]

The possible mechanisms underlying the postingestive inhibitory action of aspartame are discussed elsewhere.[23,27] In relation to the present discussion, however, the importance of this finding is that it helps explain some of the complexity of the data on aspartame and human appetite. In a variety of studies, aspartame has been found to bring about an increase, a decrease,

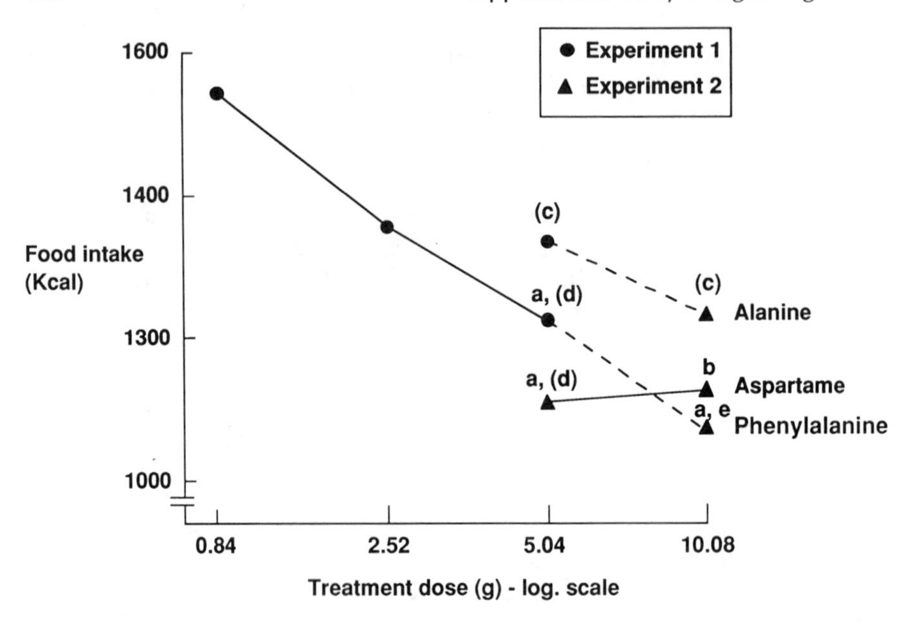


**FIGURE 1.** Effect of phenylalanine, alanine, and aspartame on food intake in men. Plotted from the data of Ryan-Harshman and colleagues.[25,26] Superscripts denote treatments which are significantly different (or nearly so): a = $p$ <0.02, b = $p$ <0.05, (c) = $p$ <0.1, compared with 0.84 g phenylalanine; (d) = $p$ <0.1, compared with 5.04 g alanine; $e$ = $p$ <0.02, compared with 10.08 g alanine. All analyses were conducted using two-tail, paired, or unpaired $t$ tests as appropriate (subjects used in Experiment 1 were different from those used in Experiment 2).

**TABLE 2**
**Effects of Aspartame on Subsequent Food Intake (vs. Unsweetened Control)[a]**

| | Sweetness | Postingestive action | Net effect |
|---|---|---|---|
| Food | + | 0 | + |
| Drink | + | – / – – | 0 / – |
| Capsule | 0 | – – | – – |

[a] Key: +, stimulation; 0, no effect; –, inhibition; – –, strong inhibition.

or no net change in food intake (see above).[1] Table 2 indicates how these results can arise from the interaction of the postingestive and taste-stimulated effects of aspartame as modified by its mode of administration. We suggest that when aspartame is consumed along with nutrients in a food there is a stimulation of appetite due to sweetness, but little or no postingestive inhibitory effect because the presence of the nutrients slows the rate of delivery of aspartame to its proposed site of action in the duodenum.[22,27] The net effect is a weakening of the satiating effect of the preload — test meal food intake was significantly greater following consumption of aspartame-sweetened yogurts compared with an equicaloric unsweetened yogurts (Table 1).[11,12]

On the other hand, a zero-calorie drink sweetened with aspartame will empty relatively rapidly from the stomach. Therefore the inhibitory postingestive effect of aspartame can be expected, at least partly, to offset the stimulatory effect of sweetness, resulting in no net change or a small reduction in intake. We have found that food intake is somewhat reduced after drinking aspartame-sweetened water compared with plain water,[9,22] a result also reported by other workers. Birch et al.,[28] for example, observed a reduction in food intake following the consumption of an aspartame-sweetened drink, although only when there was a delay of 30 or 60 min between consumption of the drink and the start of the test meal, and not when the drink immediately preceded the meal. This is an important finding because it indicates that the inhibition of intake by aspartame was not due to its sensory effects, that is sensory satiety, since this would predict that the strongest effect would be seen in the no delay condition.

In summary, Table 2 indicates that we expect the effects of aspartame to differ according to whether it is provided in a food or a drink. It also indicates that aspartame reduces food intake most clearly when the stimulatory action of sweetness is bypassed, as in the studies examining the effects of capsulated aspartame.[22,23]

A further aspect of the effects of aspartame concerns the increases in ratings of subjective hunger and desire to eat that have been observed following, for example, the consumption of aspartame-sweetened drinks[8,9] or after chewing aspartame-sweetened gum.[13] The later result follows directly from Table 2, since chewing aspartame gum will strongly stimulate sweet taste receptors without the ingestion of significant amounts of aspartame. Originally, the findings that the consumption of an aspartame-sweetened drink led to an increase in subjective hunger followed by a decrease in food intake were harder to reconcile.[9] However, our recent studies show that there is little or no decrease in self-reported hunger following the administration of capsulated aspartame.[22,23] This suggests that the reduction in food intake seen in these studies is due primarily to an intensification of intrameal satiety. Therefore, the apparently paradoxical effects of consuming a zero-calorie drink sweetened with aspartame probably arise because the postingestive action of aspartame antagonizes only the effect of sweetness on food intake, and does not modify the sweetness-induced increase in preprandial hunger.

## V. CONCLUSIONS

From the discussion above it is clear that laboratory research on sweeteners and appetite has produced a complex series of findings from which, nonetheless, some important principles are beginning to emerge. Both the sensory and postingestive effects of sweeteners can influence appetite. Sweet taste can stimulate hunger and food intake, and the postingestive effects of calories can suppress appetite. Consequently, intense (low calorie) sweeteners have low satiating power compared with sugars and other carbohydrates. In addition, this work has demonstrated that intense sweeteners can have direct postingestive effects — given their potent sensory effects, it is perhaps not so surprising that these substances also appear to act on other physiological systems. Intense sweeteners have, therefore, provided a valuable experimental tool for examining appetite mechanisms. In turn, the results of this work are relevant to the use of intense sweeteners as an aid to dietary control. One conclusion must be that the incorporation of intense sweeteners into the diet will not lead "automatically" to a reduction in energy intake or body weight. On the other hand, any beneficial effects of these substances will be determined by many additional factors that probably cannot be modeled adequately in the laboratory. Thus the efficacy of intense sweeteners, and low-calorie products in general, will depend on informed decision, strong motivation, and the ability to comply with recommendations to adjust life-style (calorie intake, eating profile, physical exercise, etc.). Low-calorie products provide consumers with the opportunity to incorporate one type of dietary adjustment into their life-style. The existence and consumption of low-calorie products per se are not sufficient to ensure weight loss or weight maintenance. Future studies should attempt to address these issues as well as to further elucidate the psychobiological effects of sweeteners.

## REFERENCES

1. Rolls, B. J., Effects of intense sweeteners on hunger, food intake, and body weight: a review, *Am. J. Clin. Nutr.*, 53, 872, 1991.
2. Brala, P.M., and Hagen, R. L., Effects of sweetness perception and caloric value of a preload on short-term intake, *Physiol. Behav.*, 30, 1, 1983.
3. Mattes, R. D., Effects of aspartame and sucrose on hunger and energy intake in humans, *Physiol. Behav.*, 47, 1037, 1990.

4. Rolls, B. J., Hetherington, M., and Jacobs, L. S., Comparison of the effects of aspartame and sucrose on appetite and food intake, *Appetite,* 11(Suppl. 1), 62, 1988.
5. Rolls, B. J., Sweetness and satiety. In: *Sweetness,* J. Dobbing, Ed. Springer-Verlag, Heidelberg, 1987, 161.
6. Foltin, R. W., Fischman, M. W., Moran, T. H., Rolls, B. J., and Kelly, T. H., Caloric compensation for lunches varying in fat and carbohydrate content by humans in a residential laboratory, *Am. J. Clin. Nutr.,* 52, 969, 1990.
7. Rolls, B. J., Hetherington, M., and Burley, V. J., The specificity of satiety: the influence of foods of different macronutrient content on the development of satiety, *Physiol. Behav.,* 43, 145, 1988.
8. Blundell, J. E., and Hill, A. J., Paradoxical effects of an intense sweetener (aspartame) on appetite, *Lancet.,* 1, 1092, 1986.
9. Rogers, P. J., Carlyle, J.-A., Hill, A. J., and Blundell, J. E., Uncoupling sweet taste and calories: comparison of the effects of glucose and three intense sweeteners on hunger and food intake, *Physiol. Behav.,* 43, 547, 1988.
10. Rogers, P. J., and Blundell, J. E., Separating the actions of sweetness and calories: effects of saccharin and carbohydrates on hunger and food intake in human subjects, *Physiol. Behav.,* 45, 1093, 1989.
11. Rogers, P. J., Lambert, T. C., Alikhanizadeh, L. A., and Blundell, J. E., Intense sweeteners and appetite: responses of informed and uninformed subjects consuming food sweetened with aspartame or sugar, *Int. J. Obes.,* 14, 105, 1990.
12. Blundell, J. E., and Rogers, P. J., Carbohydrates and satiety, *C-H-O: Int. Dialogue Carbohydr.,* 2, 1, 1991.
13. Tordoff, M. G., and Alleva, A. M., Oral stimulation with aspartame stimulates hunger, *Physiol. Behav.,* 47, 555, 1990.
14. Tordoff, M. G., and Reed, D. R., Sham-feeding sucrose and corn oil stimulates food intake in rats, *Appetite,* 17, 97, 1991.
15. Blundell, J. E., Rogers P. J., and Hill, A. J., Uncoupling sweet taste and calories: methodological aspects of laboratory studies on appetite control, *Appetite,* 11 (Suppl. 1), 54, 1988.
16. Rogers, P. J., and Blundell, J. E., Evaluation of the influence of intense sweeteners on the short-term control of appetite and caloric intake — a psychobiological approach. In: *Progress in Sweeteners,* T. H. Grenby, Ed. Elsevier Applied Science, London, 1989, chap. 10.
17. Flatt, J. P., Importance of nutrient balance in body weight regulation, *Diabetes Metab. Rev.,* 6, 571, 1988.
18. Schutz, Y., Flatt J. P., and Jequier, E., Failure of dietary fat intake to promote fat oxidation: a factor favoring the development of obesity, *Am. J. Clin. Nutr.,* 50, 307, 1989.
19. Porikos, K. P., Hesser, M. F., and Van Itallie, T. B., Caloric regulation in normal-weight men maintained on a palatable diet of conventional foods, *Physiol. Behav.,* 29, 293, 1982.
20. Tremblay, A., Ploure, G., Despre, J. P., and Bouchard, C., Impact of dietary fat content and fat oxidation on energy intake in humans, *Am. J. Clin. Nutr.,* 49, 799, 1989.

21. Beaton, G. H., Tarasuk, V., and Anderson, G. H., Estimation of possible impact of non-caloric fat and carbohydrate substitutes on macronutrient intake in the human, *Appetite,* 19, 87, 1992.
22. Rogers, P. J., Pleming, H. C., and Blundell, J. E., Aspartame consumed without tasting inhibits hunger and food intake, *Physiol. Behav.,* 47, 1239, 1990.
23. Rogers, P. J., Keedwell, P., and Blundell, J. E., Further analysis of the short-term inhibition of food intake in humans by the dipeptide L-aspartyl-L-phenylalanine methyl ester, *Physiol. Behav.,* 49, 739, 1991.
24. Rodin, J., Effects of pure sugar vs. mixed starch fructose loads on food intake, *Appetite,* 17, 213, 1991.
25. Ryan-Harshman, M., Leiter, L. A., and Anderson, G. H., Phenylalanine and aspartame fail to alter feeding behaviour, mood and arousal in men, *Physiol. Behav.,* 39, 247, 1987.
26. Ryan-Harshman, M., Mealtime food intake and behavior of normal weight adult males: effects of phenylalanine and aspartame, Ph.D. thesis, the University of North Carolina at Greensboro, 1987.
27. Rogers, P. J., and Blundell, J. E., Satiation induced by the dipeptide L-aspartyl-L-phenylalanine methyl ester (aspartame): possible involvement of CCK. In: *Multiple Cholecystokinin Receptors: Progress Towards CNS Therapeutic Targets,* C. T. Dourish, S. J. Cooper, S. D. Iversen, and L. L. Iversen, Eds. Oxford University Press, Oxford, 1992, chap. 28.
28. Birch, L. L., McPhee, L., and Sullivan, S., Children's food intake following drinks sweetened with aspartame: time course effects, *Physiol. Behav.,* 45, 387, 1988.

# 9 Sweeteners, Food Intake, and Selection

Richard M. Black and G. Harvey Anderson

## I. INTRODUCTION

The role of caloric and noncaloric (or high-intensity) sweeteners in influencing food intake and food selection has led to considerable debate in both scientific and public fora. Yet the two fundamental questions surrounding this issue remain unanswered. First, is the effect of a caloric sweetener on food intake and selection different from that of an intense (low- or noncaloric) sweetener? and second, if a difference exists, is this difference predictable based solely on the presence or absence of energy content?

In recent years many have attempted to identify the role of sweeteners on food intake, separate from the energy content of the food or drink containing the sweetener, leading to heated discussion around the most suitable experimental strategy. Some advocate that when assessing the effect of sweeteners on appetite, the base food without any added sweetener should also be assessed.[1] However, others argue strongly that such a condition (which might be represented by an unflavored, unsweetened gelatin) is wholly unnatural, most likely unpalatable, and so would probably yield meaningless information.[2] Not surprisingly, both experimental approaches are currently being used.

The role of intense sweeteners in the diet, and their potential benefit with regard to food intake and health, remains to be determined. In fact, much of the debate over the comparative benefit of caloric vs. intense sweeteners arises from the successful development of the high-intensity sweetener aspartame (APM), now widely used in the food supply. Initially, the development of high-intensity sweeteners was motivated by the erroneous perception that sweetness together with calories accounted for excessive food intake. This development took advantage of the "sweetness without calories", suggesting that excessive energy intake could be avoided through the use of these sweeteners. However, despite numerous studies of the role of intense sweeteners in weight control,[3-8] this putative benefit remains unproven.

0-8493-4466-2/94/$0.00+$.50

In the following, we review the effect of sweeteners on food intake and selection first by examining sugar consumption data, because this is relevant to addressing the perception that sweetness and calories lead to excessive energy intake, and second by examining current research describing the effect of caloric and noncaloric sweeteners on food intake.

## II. SWEETENER CONSUMPTION

During the early 1970s, it was widely stated that caloric sweetener consumption (i.e., free sugars, including sucrose, high fructose corn syrups, etc.) was excessive, had increased in the past 50 years, and directly contributed to the excessive energy intake and adverse health status in a large proportion of the North American population.[9] This view influenced expert committees charged with setting dietary guidelines, with the result that many countries set goals for maximum sugar intake in the range of 10 to 12% of dietary energy. Interestingly, this recommended range is very close to our best estimate of average sugar consumption by individuals (in contrast to that which is available). The perception that sugar intake should be reduced most likely arises from the misunderstood data on the national consumption of sugars (Figure 1).[9] Consumption estimates have always been equated with estimates of availability, which is approximately 127 lb/year/individual (57.7 kg/year/individual). However, sugar is used in many more ways than simply as a sweetener for coffee or a morning cereal. There are a large number of food processes that lead to its fermentation (e.g., bread making, distilling), it is often wasted, or it may be used in one of many nonhuman applications (e.g., pet food). Therefore, disappearance or availability data provide a gross overestimate of actual sugar consumption. The most thorough analysis of consumption based on dietary survey data suggest that only one-third of that available (roughly 43 lb or 20 kg/year) is consumed by the average individual. This represents approximately 10 to 12% of dietary energy, which is in line with dietary recommendations. So there is little need for a stated dietary *goal*, since a *goal* generally implies a change in behavior is required.

In recent dietary guidelines, both Canada[10] and the United States[11] have refrained from setting national goals for sugar intake, and no longer suggest that a population reduction in the intake of caloric sweeteners is necessary. Rather, published guidelines suggest that sugars be used in moderation. This is not a universally accepted recommendation, though. The World Health Organization (WHO) has advised that the added sugar intake fall in the range of 0 to 10% of total dietary energy.[12] This implies that the 10 to 12% of dietary energy as added sugar typical of the average North American individual should be reduced, and that nutritionally healthy and practical diets can be achieved with no added sugar. There is no evidence in support of (or contrary to) either contention.

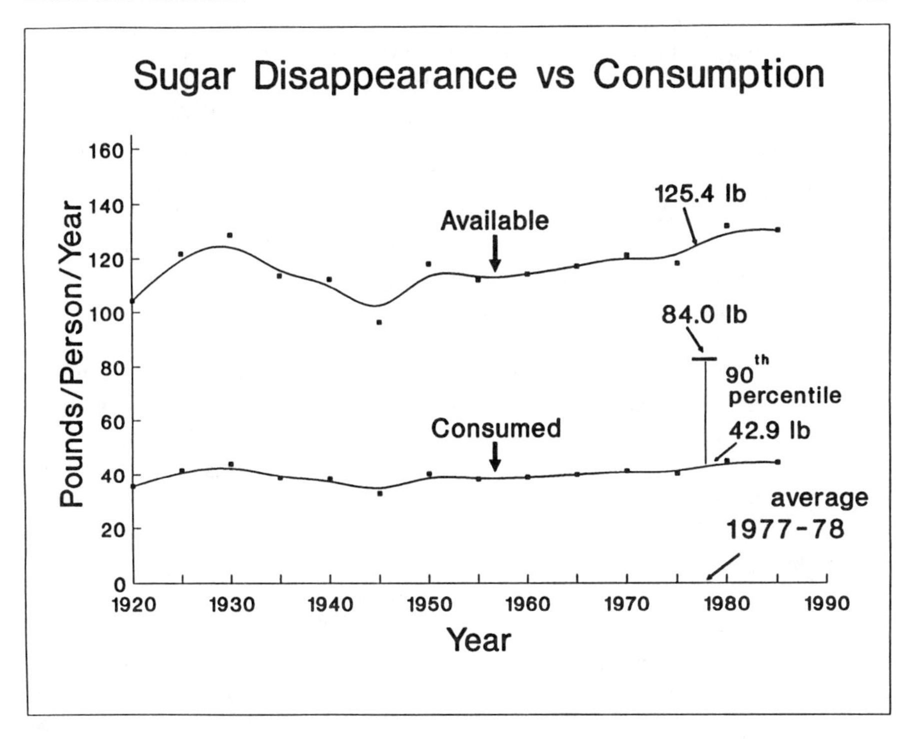


**FIGURE 1.** A comparison of the amount of sugar available to the amount consumed *as sugar*. The line depicting consumption is extrapolated from data recorded in 1977 and 1978, and so may not be a precise representation of consumption, but nonetheless serves to illustrate the dramatic difference between availability and consumption.

From Figure 1, it can be seen that free sugar availability has not increased in any significant way over the past 50 years. One might predict, therefore, that consumption has also been relatively constant and therefore does not account for the increased risk of chronic disease seen over the same time period.[13] Specifically, it is clear that the increased incidence of obesity has occurred independently of the quantitative consumption of sugar. These data might also be interpreted to suggest that sweetness does not by itself generate an excessive energy intake. Thus in the following, we present data relevant to this interpretation.

## III. SWEETENERS AND FOOD INTAKE: A MATTER OF CALORIES?

### A. Caloric Sweeteners

While there have been numerous studies on the effects of a caloric preload on subsequent food intake,[14] there is remarkably little literature bearing on the effect of nutritive sweeteners on appetite, and whether calories from these sugars are seen by the appetite regulatory systems in the same way as other carbohydrate energy. Most studies have observed no effect of a nutritive sweetener on the food intake of adults at a meal given 40 min,[15] 30 or 60 min,[16] or 60 min[17] after the sweetened drink is consumed. However, if the calories from sugar consumed in the drink are added to the calories consumed during the test meal in these studies, there is often a significant increase in total calories consumed[15,16] (see Canty and Chan[17]). These short-term studies hint at the possibility that added sugar in the diet might lead to an increased energy intake, but do not take into account the possibility that energy intake adjustments may take place at later meals. Based on an extensive literature review, Glinsman et al.[13] concluded that added sugars in the diet do not lead to a positive energy balance except insofar as they are part of a diet that is excessive in terms of energy intake in the first place. This in turn suggests that sugar energy is in no way different from energy provided by any other form of metabolizable carbohydrates and that sucrose should suppress appetite in proportion to its energy content and similar to other carbohydrates.

To begin to develop an understanding of the acute effects of sugar on food intake, both quantitative (i.e., caloric) and time relationships to the meal need to be described. Both of these factors will impact on any compensatory response, and so must be considered when conclusions are drawn describing the effect of the preload on energy adjustment in a subsequent meal.

We have examined the effect of sugar on the appetite and food intake of children.[18] A cherry flavored Kool-Aid drink was used as a vehicle in providing 9- and 10-year-old children 0, 45, or 90 g of sugar in a 300 ml volume (0, 180, and 360 kcal, respectively). Consuming the sugar-sweetened drink significantly altered both the total food intake and the food choice of these children at a buffet lunch meal offered 30 min later. The children compensated for 68 and 63% of the calories consumed in the 180 and 360 kcal preloads, respectively, reducing their lunch-time intake on average by 122 and 227 kcal. So although the children did not fully compensate for 100% of the calories contained in the drink, the sugar calories clearly had an impact on food intake regulatory mechanisms (Figure 2).

Somewhat more surprising were the food selections made by the children, and the change in these selections after each of the caloric preloads. When the children consumed the unsweetened Kool-Aid, cookies were the most preferred food (as measured by total energy intake). However, when 45 g of sugar was consumed in the drink, cookies dropped in preference leaving bread as the most preferred food. In the 90 g sugar condition, preference for cookies declined even further, being surpassed by meats in addition to breads and cakes. Thus the preload of sugar not only reduced

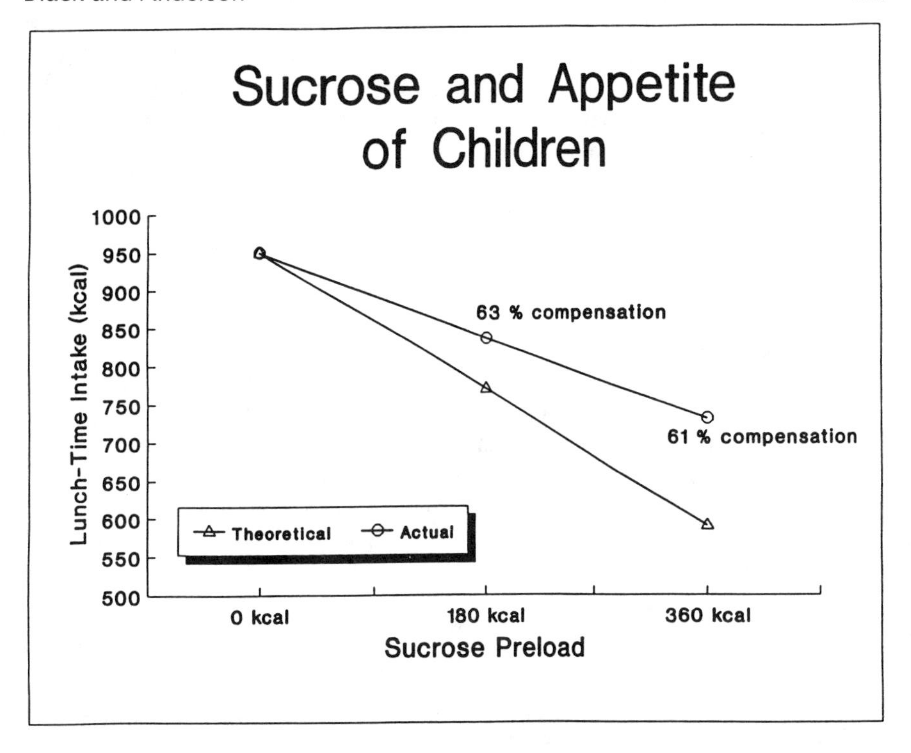


**FIGURE 2.** Theoretical and actual lunch-time energy intakes are shown, following consumption of a preload containing 0, 180, or 360 kcal 30 min prior to lunch. The theoretical line represents expected intake if the subjects compensated fully for the calories consumed in the preload. Actual compensation is the reduction in energy intake from the 0 kcal condition.

total energy intake, but also reduced the intake of sweet foods as indicated by a decrease in the preference for and consumption of cookies, perhaps as a result of the sensory-specific satiety as proposed by Rolls and colleagues.[19]

In both this[20] and a previous study,[21] we observed that a preload of sugar given 90 min before the meal had no effect on lunch-time food intake or food selection. Taken together, the results of these two studies demonstrate that the acute appetite effect of a caloric preload is time dependent, but the results do not provide any information on energy intake compensation occurring later in the day as observed by Birch and colleagues.[22]

The earlier failures to demonstrate an effect of a sugar preload on the appetite of adults[15,16] suggest that age may also be a factor. Daily energy intake of children appears to be more tightly regulated than that of an adult, with a coefficient of variation averaging 10% in children[22] and 30% in adults[23] (though this may be due in part to an overall lower energy intake in children). Given the tighter regulation of daily energy intake, we might predict that a child will more precisely compensate at a test meal for the calories ingested in a preload. In fact, Birch et al.[22] reported a tendency in children for meal size to be negatively correlated with the size of the previous meal. That is, the children are compensating for the calories consumed at the previous meal.

These studies show that at least in children, sugar calories can provide appetite signals and alter food intake. However, the data do not show if the impact is the same as for other carbohydrates and, unfortunately, comparative data are not available in the literature.

## B. High-Intensity Sweeteners

The widespread demand for intense sweeteners has been created from the simple assumption that intense sweeteners will help reduce caloric intake by decreasing sugar intake, and so help weight management. However, in recent years the converse hypothesis, that consuming intense sweeteners may *increase* appetite and possibly energy intake, has drawn a great deal of interest.

### 1. High-Intensity Sweeteners and Reduced Energy Intake

As indicated earlier, high-intensity sweeteners are primarily distinguished from sugars by their absence of calories. Although some have hypothesized that the metabolic byproducts of APM may have specific physiologic consequences, none has yet been demonstrated. For example, it has been suggested that the phenylalanine component of APM may stimulate the endogenous release of cholecystokinin thereby promoting satiety. In addition, it has been suggested that phenylalanine may alter brain levels of the catecholamines involved in the control of feeding, for which it serves as a precursor.[24]

On the other hand, many studies have shown that replacing the caloric sweeteners in a diet with a low or noncaloric (intense) sweetener results in little if any change in energy intake.[8,25-27] Subjects consume a larger volume of food when the caloric density is reduced and so maintain energy intake.[6,28] An exception to this general statement appears to be provided by the studies of Porikos and colleagues wherein the energy intakes of volunteer subjects were measured before, during, and after the covert substitution of aspartame for sugar, which made up 25% of the total dietary calories. While the data from these studies suggest that using an intense sweetener in place of sugar can lead to a reduction in food intake (Porikos et al. report a sustained intake reduction of approximately 15%), several alternative explanations for the reduced energy intake have been proposed.[3-5]

First, in these studies the subjects were gaining weight during the baseline period on sugar. When aspartame was used in the diet, the reduction in caloric intake stabilized weight but did not result in a weight loss. When sugar was reintroduced, once again weight began to increase. This observation suggests that the subjects were likely overeating during baseline, possibly because of the wide array of food presented to them on an *ad libitum* basis, and that the caloric dilution may have reduced intake by making it difficult (if not impossible) to consume sufficient bulk to maintain the previously elevated intake. For instance, assuming an average caloric density of 1500 kcal/kg food,[29] a person consuming 2500 kcal/day would be eating 1.8 kg of food. Maintenance of energy intake during the dilution period of the Porikos study would have required a daily food intake of approximately 3 kg, a near doubling of food intake.

Second, all subjects experienced a sugar/aspartame/sugar rotation in the diet, and so there are no data on subjects exposed to an aspartame/sugar/aspartame rotation. This makes it difficult to distinguish between the impact of familiarity with the diet and the role of the sweetener in the diet. For example, it could be argued that there was significant overconsumption, even hyperphagia, during the first 3 to 6 days of the study (the duration of the initial sugar period) due to the novelty of the diet. What might the intake have been if aspartame were used as the sweetener during the first 6 days? Might intake have been elevated during this time? Unfortunately, the data do not directly address this issue.

In summary, the effect on food intake and energy balance of replacing sugar with high-intensity sweeteners to produce food low in energy density remains unresolved. In the longer term, it seems likely that energy balance mechanisms will compensate for the casual use of such products by the population. However, it may be that the use of products containing high-intensity sweeteners will reduce consumption of sugar-containing foods and have a tendency to shift food selection toward high-fat foods, thus replacing energy intake and increasing fat intake relative to total dietary energy.[30]

### 2. High-Intensity Sweeteners and Increased Appetite

The role of intense sweeteners in the diet, especially as they are used in low-calorie beverages, has stirred considerable controversy over the last 6 years following the report of Blundell and Hill[31] that aspartame-sweetened beverages lead to an increase in subjective appetite and possibly food intake. Blundell and colleagues have hypothesized that this appetite increase is a direct result of experiencing a sweet taste in the absence of any calories.[32] They and others[33-35] hypothesize that sweet taste generally predicts calories, and that when a sweet taste is experienced subtle changes in metabolism might occur that prepare the body for these incoming calories. When these calories are not forthcoming, the person experiences an increase in appetite.

Many attempts to replicate the report of Blundell and Hill[31] have failed (see Rolls[36] for a review) with only one exception. Recently, we also observed that APM added to water increases subjective appetite.[37] Young adult male subjects consumed 340 mg of APM in 280 ml of mineral water. An increase in appetite was reported that lasted from 20 to 30 min, compared to an unsweetened control (Figure 3). While the APM drink had no impact on energy intake or food selection measured 60 min after the drink, in effect we were providing the food to the subjects a full 30 min *after* the increase in appetite had disappeared. It might be very informative to observe food intake during that time when subjective appetite is increased. Interestingly, despite the APM-induced increase in subjective appetite, the subjective appeal of most foods actually decreased following ingestion of the APM drink.

The application of this observation to normal use of aspartame in commercial drinks seems unlikely however. We studied the effect of APM-sweetened diet soft drinks on the subjective appetite and food intake of young adult males, and found that compared to a carbonated mineral water control (Perrier), 280 ml of the diet soda had no effect on appetite, food intake, or food selection.[34,35] Although 560 ml of the diet soda suppressed appetite for the next 30 to 45 min, there were no effects on food intake at the meal presented 60 min after the drink. We[34,35] and others[2] have pointed out in the past that APM-sweetened water is an unfamiliar stimulus, one that is unlikely to be encountered outside of the laboratory. In contrast, it would be difficult if not impossible to find someone who had not experienced an aspartame-sweetened diet soda or other aspartame-sweetened nonalcoholic drink. Those studies unable to detect an effect of APM on appetite have used a familiar drink.[15,17,34-36] Thus it is possible that the novelty of the APM-sweetened water contributes in some manner to the increased appetite.

Rogers et al.[38,39] reported that ingesting APM without taste (in a gelatin capsule) leads to a decrease in appetite and food intake. While they have suggested that the decrease might be due to the postingestive effects of the phenlyalanine component of APM, this seems unlikely as they have not been able to replicate this effect with the administration of phenylalanine alone.[38] In two separate experiments, we have examined the effects on appetite of consuming APM without taste, i.e., in the form of a pill. In the first study, subjects consumed 5 or 10 g of APM with no significant change in appetite or food intake.[40] While it has been suggested that the number of pills consumed to achieve these levels of APM intake was excessive,[39] we have recently studied appetite and food intake following ingestion of 340 mg of APM in two gelatin capsules. Once again, we observed no change in appetite or food intake.[34,35] Finally, while we have been unable to detect any decrease in appetite following ingestion of APM pills, it might be argued that the suppression in appetite we observed after the consumption of 560 ml of a diet

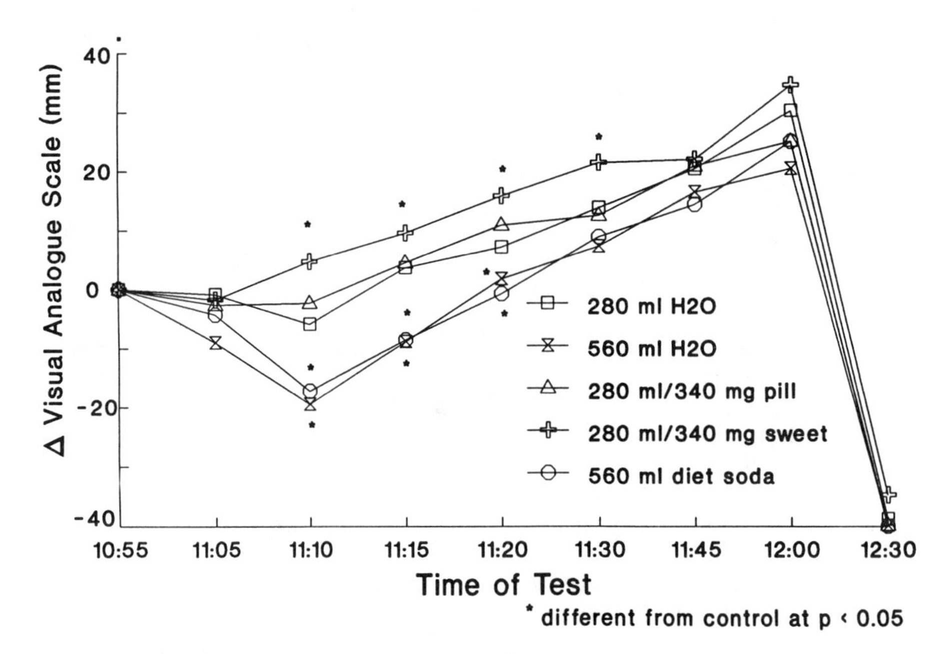


**FIGURE 3.** Subjective measures of Desire to Eat for subjects following consumption of preloads as indicated. Note that consuming 340 mg of APM as a sweetener in mineral water increases subjective appetite, while consuming the same amount in two gelatin capsules (labeled "pill" in the figure) does not. Also, 560 ml of mineral water reduces subjective appetite to the same extent as 560 ml of APM-sweetened diet soda.

soda (containing 340 mg APM) was due to the APM content of the drink and not the volume. However, this seems unlikely since we have been able to demonstrate that 560 ml of carbonated mineral water suppresses appetite to the same extent, and for the same duration, as 560 ml of diet soda.[34,35]

## IV. SUMMARY

The role of sugars and sweeteners in appetite control remains poorly defined, but there is no evidence that excessive intake is a consequence of either. Furthermore, there is no convincing data to disprove the hypothesis that the effects of high-intensity sweeteners on food intake are primarily distinguished from sugar by their absence of calories, and not by any metabolic sequelae or physiological effects resulting from ingesting sweetness in the absence of calories. The majority of studies indicate that when high-intensity sweeteners are substituted for sugar in foods and beverages, food intake is adjusted to compensate for the reduction in caloric density. The increase in appetite following ingestion of APM in water has not yet been proven to apply to familiar beverages. Therefore we must be cautious at this point in any attempts to extend this beyond the confines of the laboratory.

## REFERENCES


1. Blundell, J. E., Rogers, P. J., and Hill, A. J., Uncoupling sweetness and calories: methodological aspects of laboratory studies on appetite control, *Appetite,* 11 (Suppl.), 54, 1988.
2. Rolls, B. J., Human studies of sweeteners and intake, *Appetite,* 11 (Suppl.), 92, 1988.
3. Porikos, K. P., Booth, G., and Van Itallie, T. B., Effect of covert nutritive dilution on the spontaneous intake of obese individuals: a pilot study, *Am. J. Clin. Nutr.,* 30, 1638, 1977.
4. Porikos, K. P., Hesser, M. F., and Van Itallie, T. B., Caloric regulation in normal weight men maintained on a palatable diet of conventional foods, *Physiol. Behav.,* 29, 293, 1982.
5. Porikos, K. P., and Pi-Sunyer, F. X., Regulation of food intake in human obesity: studies with caloric dilution and exercise, *Clin. Endocrinol. Metab.,* 13, 547, 1984.
6. Foltin, R. W., Fischman, M. W., Emurian, C. S., and Rachlinski, J. J., Compensation for caloric dilution in humans given unrestricted access to food in a residential laboratory, *Appetite,* 10, 13, 1988.
7. Kanders, B. S., Kowalchuk, M., Lavin, P., and Blackburn, G. L., Do aspartame (APM) sweetened foods and beverages aid in long-term control of body weight?, *Am. J. Clin. Nutr.,* 51, 515, 1990.
8. Kanders, B. S., Lavin, P. T., Kowalchuk, M. B., Greenberg, I., and Blackburn, G. L., An evaluation of the effect of aspartame on weight loss, *Appetite,* 11 (Suppl.), 73, 1988.
9. Anderson, G. H., Sugar consumption: are dietary guidelines needed?, *J. Can. Diet. Assoc.,* 50, 229, 1989.
10. Health and Welfare Canada. *Nutrition Recommendations: The Report of the Scientific Review Committee.* Canadian Government Publishing Centre, Ottawa, 1990.
11. United States Department of Agriculture and Health and Human Services. *Nutrition and Your Health: Dietary Guidelines for Americans.* Washington, D.C., 1990.
12. World Health Organization (WHO). *Diet, Nutrition and the Prevention of Chronic Diseases.* Report of a WHO Study Group. Technical Report Series 797. World Health Organization, Geneva, 1990.
13. Glinsman, W. H., Irausquin, H., and Park, Y. K., Report from FDA's Sugar Task Force, 1986. Evaluation of health aspects of sugars contained in carbohydrate sweeteners, *J. Nutr.,* 116 (Suppl. 11), S1, 1986.

14. Rolls, B. J., Hetherington, M., and Laster, L. J., Comparison of the effects of aspartame and sucrose on food intake, *Appetite,* 11 (Suppl.), 62, 1988.
15. Rodin, J., Comparative effects of fructose, aspartame, glucose and water beverages on calorie and macronutrient intake, *Am. J. Clin. Nutr.,* 51, 428, 1990.
16. Rolls, B. J., Kim, S., and Federoff, I. C., Effects of drinks sweetened with sucrose or aspartame on hunger, thirst and food intake in men, *Physiol. Behav.,* 48, 19, 1990.
17. Canty, D. J., and Chan, M. M., Effects of consumption of caloric vs. noncaloric sweet drinks on indices of hunger and food consumption in normal adults, *Am. J. Clin. Nutr.,* 53, 1159, 1991.
18. Crombie, C., Anderson, G. H., Leiter, L. A., Zlotkin, S., Schacher, R., Tanaka, P., and Black, R. M., Effect of sucrose preload on subjective measures of appetite and food intake in children, *Proc. 33rd Ann. Meet. Can. Fed. Biolog. Sci.,* (Abstr.), 127, 1990.
19. Rolls, B. J., Hetherington, M., Burley, S. J., and Duijvenvoorde, P. M., Changing hedonic response to food during and after a meal. In: *Interaction of the Chemical Senses with Nutrition,* M. R. Kare, and J. G. Brand, Eds. Academic Press, New York, 1986, 247.
20. Crombie, C., Effect of a sucrose preload on food intake and subjective measures of appetite in 9 and 10 year old healthy children. Master's of Science Thesis, University of Toronto, Toronto, Canada, 1992.
21. Anderson, G. H., Saravis, S., Schacher, R., Zlotkin, S., and Leiter, L. A., Aspartame: effect on lunch-time food intake, appetite and hedonic response in children, *Appetite,* 13, 93, 1989.
22. Birch, L. L., Johnson, S. L., Andersen, G., and Peters, J. C., The variability of young children's energy intake, *N. Engl. J. Med.,* 324, 232, 1991.
23. Tarasuk, V., and Beaton, G. H., The nature and individuality of within-subject variation in energy intake, *Am. J. Clin. Nutr.,* 54, 464, 1991.
24. Anderson, G. H., and Leiter, L. A., Effects of aspartame and phenylalanine on meal-time food intake in humans, *Appetite,* 11 (Suppl.), 48, 1988.
25. Van Itallie, T. B., Yang, M. U., and Porikos, K. P., Use of aspartame to test the "Body weight set point" hypothesis, *Appetite,* 11 (Suppl.), 68, 1988.
26. Mattes, R., Effects of aspartame and sucrose on energy intake and hunger in humans, *Physiol. Behav.,* 47, 1037, 1990.
27. Mattes, R., Pierce, C. B., and Friedman, M. I., Daily caloric intake of normal-weight adults: response to changes of dietary energy density of a luncheon meal, *Am. J. Clin. Nutr.,* 48, 214, 1988.
28. Foltin, R. W., Fischman, M. W., Moran, T. H., Rolls, B. J., and Kelly, T. H., Caloric compensation for lunches varying in fat and carbohydrate content by humans in a residential laboratory, *Am. J. Clin. Nutr.,* 52, 969, 1990.
29. Kendal, A., Levitsky, D. A., Strupp. B. J., and Lissner, L., Weight loss on a low-fat diet: consequence of the imprecision of the control of food intake in humans, *Am. J. Clin. Nutr.,* 53, 1124, 1991.
30. Beaton, G. H., Tarasuk, V., and Anderson, G. H., Estimation of possible impact of non-caloric fat and carbohydrate substitutes on macronutrient intake in the human, *Appetite,* 19, 87–103, 1992.

31. Blundell, J. E., and Hill, A. J., Paradoxical effects of an intense sweetener (aspartame) on appetite, *Lancet,* 1, 1092, 1986.
32. Rogers, P. J., Carlyle, J., Hill, A. J., and Blundell, J. E., Uncoupling sweet taste and calories: comparison of the effects of glucose and three intense sweeteners on hunger and food intake, *Physiol. Behav.,* 43, 547, 1988.
33. Tordoff, M. G., and Friedman, M. I., Drinking saccharin increases food intake and preference. IV. Cephalic phase and metabolic factors, *Appetite,* 12, 37, 1989.
34. Black, R. M., Leiter, L. A., and Anderson G. H., Aspartame sweetened soft drinks: volume, not aspartame, is responsible for appetite suppression, *FASEB J.,* 5 (5) (Abstr.), 5472, 1991.
35. Black, R. M., Tanaka, P., Leiter, L. A., and Anderson. G. H., Soft drinks with aspartame: effect on subjective hunger, food selection, and food intake of young adult males, *Physiol. Behav.,* 49, 803, 1991.
36. Rolls, B. J., Effects of intense sweeteners on hunger, food intake, and body weight: a review, *Am. J. Clin. Nutr.,* 53, 872, 1991.
37. Black, R. M., Leiter, L. A., and Anderson, G. H., Aspartame and water: short term enhancement and suppression of subjective appetite but not food intake, *J. Cell. Biochem.,* 16(B) (Abstr.), WB100, 1992.
38. Rogers, P. J., Pleming, H. C., and Blundell, J. E., Aspartame ingested without tasting inhibits hunger and food intake, *Physiol. Behav.,* 47, 1239, 1990.
39. Rogers, P. J., Keedwell, P., and Blundell, J. E., Further analysis of the short term inhibition of food intake in humans by the dipeptide L-aspartyl-L-phenylalanine methyl ester (aspartame), *Physiol. Behav.,* 49, 739, 1991.
40. Ryan-Harshman, M., Leiter, L. A., and Anderson, G. H., Phenylalanine and aspartame fail to alter feeding behavior, mood and arousal in men, *Physiol. Behav.,* 39, 247, 1987.

# 10 Human Preferences for Sugar and Fat

**Adam Drewnowski**

## I. INTRODUCTION

The typical American diet is composed of two principal ingredients: sugar and fat. While fat contributes 38% of total calories to the average diet, simple sugars, both natural and added, account for a further 22% of the daily caloric intake.[1-3] Although a high-fat diet that is low in complex carbohydrates is generally viewed as unhealthy,[3,4] past attempts to modify dietary behavior of individuals and groups have met with limited success. Sweet foods are as popular as ever, and despite repeated recommendations to reduce dietary fat content,[3,4] fat consumption remains high as consumers have simply learned to replace one fat source with another.[5]

Evident human appetites for sugar (a carbohydrate) and fat have led to suggestions that macronutrient consumption is directly mediated by the central nervous system. For example, recent literature on nutrition and brain function has been dominated by reports of "carbohydrate cravings".[6-8] A centrally mediated appetite or selective "craving" for carbohydrate-rich foods has been touted as a major contributing factor in human obesity.[8] In this view, a deficiency of a central neurotransmitter serotonin, said to characterize most obese people, reportedly leads them to select carbohydrates as meals or snacks even though other foods are available.[6,7,9] Such "carbohydrate cravings" have reputedly been observed among 90% of obese patients,[9,10] and excessive carbohydrate intake is said to be the major cause of human obesity syndromes.[11]

Other studies have suggested that obesity may be associated with excessive consumption of dietary fat. Dietary intake studies have shown that obese women consumed more fat calories than did lean women and had a lower dietary carbohydrate-to-fat ratio.[12] More recently, high levels of body fat have been correlated with the amount of fat in the diet[13] and with sensory preferences for high levels of fat in foods.[14]. However, no specific theory

0-8493-4466-2/94/$0.00+$.50

has yet linked the high national levels of fat consumption with central nervous system activity or with brain function.

Indeed, it is becoming increasingly clear that metabolic signals mediating food intake are strongly influenced by behavioral variables and by prior learning. In general, people prefer, select, and "crave" specific foods rather than macronutrients. It is here that taste responsiveness exerts its dominant role.

The sense of taste strongly influences food preferences and diet selection.[15-17] Taste preferences mediate the connection among metabolic status, food acceptance, and actual food consumption. On one hand, central and peripheral manipulations of metabolic status may result in altered taste responsiveness, and some metabolic events have been associated with specific food preferences or "cravings".[18-20] On the other hand, taste preferences modified by experience are the key factor in determining food acceptance and the selection of the habitual diet.[15,21] Although other behavioral and sociocultural factors also play a role in diet choice,[22,23] people respond primarily to the sensory qualities of food.

## II. THE "CARBOHYDRATE CRAVING" HYPOTHESIS

According to the "carbohydrate-craving" hypothesis, obese[6-8,11] and depressed patients,[24] bulimic women, persons with seasonal affective disorders (SAD),[25] as well as women with the premenstrual tension syndrome (PMS) all share a common underlying pathology. All are said to be characterized by a deficiency in the central neurotransmitter serotonin. Carbohydrate-rich foods consumed in the absence of protein are reputed to selectively promote the uptake of serotonin precursor tryptophan into the brain, increase the rate of serotonin synthesis, and so redress serotonin imbalance.[6-8] "Carbohydrate craving" is thus said to be the behavioral manifestation of serotonin imbalance, and a centrally mediated attempt at self-medication.[8]

The serotonin hypothesis leads to certain specific predictions. First, if "carbohydrate cravings" are indeed macronutrient-specific, then the patterns of consumption of carbohydrate-rich snacks should be the same for sweet and for nonsweet foods. According to the serotonin hypothesis, carbohydrates with a high glycemic index most effectively promote tryptophan uptake by the brain. Consequently, carbohydrates with a high glycemic index (e.g., potato starch) should be the most common object of food "cravings".[24]

Furthermore, the fat content of foods should be immaterial, with no special distinction made between potatoes and chocolate. Indeed, since

The Potato Man
Fall must really be here, because...
DING DING DING! Here comes the Potato Man!
POTATO MAN
Oh, boy! Chocolate-coated taters on a stick! Ma, can I have some money?
POTATO POP 35¢
Mmm... those mashed-potato sandwiches look pretty tempting!
SANDWICH TREAT 45¢
And look - he's got cones in yam, Idaho, or tiny red -
with your choice of topping!
JIMMIES
CHOCOLATE SAUCE
PARSLEY AND SOUR CREAM
I'll have me one of those!
See you tomorrow, Potato Man!
R. Chast

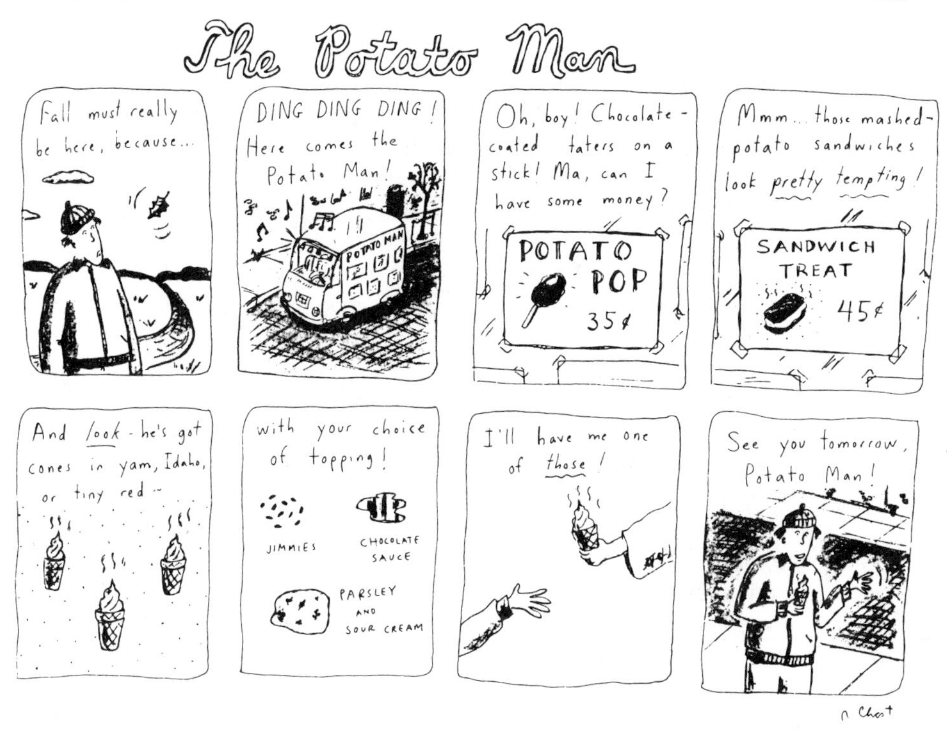

**FIGURE 1.** The spirit of the alleged "carbohydrate craving" phenomenon is captured in this drawing by R. Chast, which appeared in the October 24, 1988 issue of *The New Yorker Magazine*. (Drawing by R. Chast, © *The New Yorker Magazine,* Inc.)

carrots and potatoes appear to have a higher glycemic index than does chocolate candy,[26] potatoes rather than chocolate should be the principal object of food cravings. (Figure 1).

Unfortunately, most studies on "carbohydrate cravings" have been conducted with ice cream or chocolate[6-8,22] and not with carrots or potato starch. This methodological defect was handled by the simple expedient of classifying ice cream and chocolate as "carbohydrate-rich" foods.[6,7,27]

There are in fact some good reasons for this misconception. First, as noted above, people generally tend to think in terms of foods and not macronutrients. Many foods provide carbohydrate, protein, or fat in different amounts, and the perception of what constitutes a high-carbohydrate or a high-fat food is often a judgment that involves both psychology and nutrition. Inevitably, misclassifications abound. The very term "carbohydrate craving" coined by Paykel et al.[18] was originally described as "a ravenous appetite for a variety of sweet substances including chocolates, cake, pastry and ice cream." Since that time, both chocolate bars and a vanilla ice cream sundae with whipped cream have been described in published studies as carbohydrate-rich foods.[7,27]

The carbohydrate in such foods is generally sugar, while most of the calories are derived from fat.[28] Sensory studies have shown that sugar is often the salient attribute of sweet desserts, since it tends to mask the perception of fat, especially in solid foods.[29] Consequently, obese patients who "crave" ice cream and chocolate-covered peanuts may well describe themselves as being addicted to sugar, that is as "carbohydrate cravers".[30]

## III. THE OPIOID PEPTIDE HYPOTHESIS

Strong preferences or "cravings" for specific foods undoubtedly exist and may well be triggered by central metabolic events. However, such "cravings" are invariably influenced by the sensory qualities of food and do not appear to be macronutrient specific. The typical objects of food "cravings", at least for women, appear to be chocolate, ice cream, doughnuts, cookies, and cake.[31,32] Such foods are typically sweet and can be regarded as sugar/fat mixtures.[28]

One central mechanism that may mediate the hedonic or pleasure response to such foods involves endogenous opioid peptides. In several studies with rats and mice, the consumption of sugar and fat has been linked to the opioid peptide system.[33] Dietary studies have shown that morphine-injected animals selectively increase fat intake, while the opioid antagonist naltrexone blocks overeating induced by a palatable cafeteria diet.[34]

Opioid peptides may influence energy intakes by mediating the pleasure response to foods. Sensory preferences for sweet taste, in particular, appear to be under opioid control. It may be that opioid blockade renders palatable foods less rewarding. In studies with rats, opioid antagonists were most effective in reducing intakes of palatable sweet liquids. Conversely, morphine administration enhanced preferences for sweet taste and stimulated the intake of sweet solutions. Some investigators have proposed that the primary role of the opioid peptide system is in mediating overeating that is associated with exposure to palatable sweet or high-fat foods.[34]

Clinical studies have shown that opioid blockade reduces sensory pleasure response and the consumption of good-tasting foods. Oral doses of naltrexone reduced pleasantness ratings of glucose solutions and the acceptability of food odors.[35] Another study showed that opioid antagonist nalmefene selectively reduced intake of the most preferred foods during a lunch meal.[36] Most recently, naltrexone was shown to reduce alcohol cravings in alcoholics, thus contributing to the success of treatment.[37]

Preferences and "cravings" for sweet high-fat foods observed among obese and bulimic patients may also involve the endogenous opioid peptide system. In a recent study,[20] the opioid antagonist naloxone, opioid agonist butorphanol, and saline placebo were administered by intravenous infusion to 14 female binge eaters and 12 normal-weight controls. Eight of the binge eaters were obese. In the course of drug infusion, the subjects tasted 20 different sugar/fat mixtures and were presented with a range of snack foods of varying sugar and fat content.

Naloxone reduced taste preferences relative to baseline in both binge eaters and in controls. Total caloric intake was significantly reduced by naloxone in binge eaters though not in controls. This reduction was most marked for sweet high-fat foods such as cookies and chocolate. In contrast, the consumption of other highly preferred foods such as popcorn was not affected by naloxone. Endogenous opioid peptides may thus be involved in mediating taste preferences for and the consumption of some palatable foods, notably those rich in sugar and fat.

## IV. SENSORY PREFERENCES FOR SUGAR AND FAT

Why are sweet and fat-containing foods so popular? Preferences for sugar/fat mixtures may be a learned response acquired in early childhood.[22] Sensory preferences for sweet taste appear to be innate, and sugar often serves as the chief vehicle for introducing fat calories into the children's diet. The most familiar and preferred foods in early childhood tend to be mixtures of sugar and fat. Sweet, fat-rich desserts also serve as powerful instruments of reward: acceptable behavior is conditioned by the use of nutritional reward of sugar and fat.

Studies on sensory response to foods point to the interactive nature of pleasure response to sugar and fat.[16,17,38] Past research in this area was traditionally limited to the study of sugar solutions in water. More recent studies made use of mixtures of sucrose and liquid dairy products containing different amounts of fat.[16,17] Most recently, sensory investigations have been extended to solid sugar/fat mixtures.[29]

In early studies,[16,17] subjects were asked to rate chilled mixtures of milk, cream, and sugar on nine-point category scale. The subjects rated the perceived sweetness and fat content of the stimuli and assigned a pleasantness rating to each sample. The pleasure response to sugar/fat mixtures was a synergistic function of the two ingredients. Respondents gave low ratings to low-fat sweet stimuli (skim milk) and to unsweetened dairy products of increasing fat content. In contrast, hedonic ratings for sugar/fat mixtures were high. Similar results were obtained with other fat/sugar stimuli, including sweetened mixtures of cottage cheese and cream cheese, cake frostings, and ice cream.[29,39] In every case, maximal hedonic preferences were a combined function of both sugar and fat contents.

## V. PREFERENCES FOR SWEET AND HIGH-FAT FOODS

While some studies on the role of dietary factors in human obesity have addressed carbohydrate consumption, others have focused on the role of dietary fat. However, very few studies have systematically addressed self-reported food preferences of the obese men and women. Studies of Army personnel[40,41] suggested that overweight (mostly male) recruits selected meat dishes rather than the expected desserts. Despite many anecdotal reports of an obese "sweet tooth", clinical studies have largely failed to come up with a distinguishable pattern or an obese eating style.[42,43]

Some predictions regarding the reputed characteristics of obese "carbohydrate cravers" can be derived from the serotonin hypothesis. If a vast majority of obese individuals show evidence of "carbohydrate craving", then preferences for dietary sources of carbohydrate should be a common characteristic of human obesity syndromes. Second, given that such "cravings" are centrally mediated, the same pattern of preferences for the same carbohydrate-rich foods should be observed for both men and for women.

These predictions were tested in a recent study[32] of food preferences of a large clinical sample of 386 obese women and 93 obese men. The subjects were asked for a self-generated list of 10 favorite foods. The lists were characterized by frequent instances of foods that are major sources of fat in the typical American diet. While obese men listed mostly protein/fat sources (i.e., meat dishes) among their favorites, obese women tended to list mostly carbohydrate/fat sources (doughnuts, cookies, cake) and foods that were sweet. There was no evidence that selective preferences for a single macronutrient, carbohydrate, were a standard feature of human obesity. Rather, preferences for foods that were major nutrient sources of fat as opposed to carbohydrate appeared to be the main shared characteristic of human obesity syndromes.

Table 1 lists the top 15 food sources of carbohydrate in the U.S. diet as derived from the NHANES II survey.[42] The largest single source of carbohydrate is the category of white bread, rolls, and crackers (accounting for 15.0% of carbohydrate calories), followed by nondiet soft drinks (8.5%), and doughnuts, cookies, and cake (7.5%).

A majority (56.2%) of obese women but fewer men named at least one item from the "doughnuts, cookies, or cake" category among their 10 most preferred foods. Similarly, many more women than men listed at least one instance of white bread, rolls, or crackers (54.4%), or named ice cream (51.3%) as a favorite food. However, several of the carbohydrate sources listed were also among the major sources of fat. Such carbohydrate/fat sources as doughnuts, ice cream, white bread, pasta dishes, french fries, and

**TABLE 1**
**Obese Respondents' Preferences for Foods That Are Major Sources of Carbohydrate in the U.S. Diet**

| Rank | Description | Percent of | |
|---|---|---|---|
| | | Women ($n = 386$) | Men ($n = 93$) |
| 1. | White bread, rolls, crackers | 54.4* | 37.6 |
| 2. | Regular soft drinks | 7.3* | 1.1 |
| 3. | Doughnuts, cookies, cake | 56.2* | 39.8 |
| 4. | Sugar | 0.3 | — |
| 5. | Whole milk, milk beverages | 6.0 | 6.5 |
| 6. | French fries, fried potatoes | 14.2 | 18.3 |
| 7. | Alcoholic beverages | 4.1 | 4.3 |
| 8. | Whole wheat, dark breads | 1.6 | 1.1 |
| 9. | Orange juice | 1.0 | — |
| 10. | Potatoes, excl. fried | 29.5 | 26.9 |
| 11. | Coffee, tea | 1.8 | 2.2 |
| 12. | Spaghetti and pasta | 39.1 | 37.6 |
| 13. | Ice cream, frozen desserts | 51.3 | 49.5 |
| 14. | Fruit juices | 1.8 | 2.2 |
| 15. | Cold cereals | 3.6 | 7.5 |

* = $p < 0.05$
From Drewnowski et al.[32]

sources as doughnuts, ice cream, white bread, pasta dishes, french fries, and salty snacks were listed far more frequently than "pure" carbohydrates such as potatoes, fruit juices, or cereal.

These findings suggest, first, that preferences for carbohydrate/fat sources are far more common than preferences for "pure" carbohydrate-rich foods, and second, that preferences for sweet, high-fat dessert-type foods are far more common among women than among men.

Obese men and women did not avoid high-protein foods. In the American diet, such foods are almost invariably among the major sources of fat. As shown in Table 2 the major food sources of nutrient fat in the American diet were hamburgers, cheeseburgers, and meatloaf (7.0 of fat calories), followed by hot dogs, ham, lunch meat (6.4%), and whole milk and milk beverages (6.0%). Preferences for fat sources among obese men and women were more widespread than preferences for carbohydrate sources. Meat products figured prominently among the favorite foods, especially among

**TABLE 2**
**Obese Respondents' Preferences for Foods That Are Major Sources of Total Fat in the U.S. Diet**

| | | Percent of | |
|---|---|---|---|
| **Rank** | **Description** | **Women ($n$ = 386)** | **Men ($n$ = 93)** |
| 1. | Hamburgers, cheeseburgers, meatloaf | 18.4 | 25.8 |
| 2. | Hot dogs, ham, lunch meats | 9.3 | 25.8* |
| 3. | Whole milk, milk beverages | 6.0 | 6.5 |
| 4. | Doughnuts, cookies, cake | 56.2* | 39.8 |
| 5. | Beef steaks, roasts | 41.2 | 72.0* |
| 6. | White bread, rolls, crackers | 54.4* | 37.6 |
| 7. | Eggs | 11.7 | 23.7* |
| 8. | Cheeses, excl. cottage cheese | 37.6* | 26.9 |
| 9. | Margarine | — | — |
| 10. | Mayonnaise, salad dressings | 6.5 | 2.2 |
| 11. | Pork, incl. chops, roast | 9.1 | 10.8 |
| 12. | French fries, fried potatoes | 14.2 | 18.3 |
| 13. | Salad and cooking oils | 0.3 | 5.4* |
| 14. | Butter | 10.1 | 5.4 |
| 15. | Ice cream, frozen desserts | 51.3 | 49.5 |

* = $p < 0.05$
From Drewnowski et al.[32]

the men. As many as 72% of the men but only 41.2% of the women listed steak or roast among their favorite foods. More men than women also expressed preferences for hot dogs, bacon, sausage, and other meats.

These food preference data provide no evidence that selective "cravings" for carbohydrate-rich foods are a characteristic feature of human obesity. First, preferences for foods that were common sources of fat outnumbered listed preferences for carbohydrate-rich foods. Second, obese men and women showed very distinct food preference profiles. Men tended to list protein/fat sources (i.e., meat dishes), while women primarily selected sweet carbohydrate/fat sources (i.e., desserts).

In past studies, typically conducted with predominantly female subjects, obese women expressing preferences for cookies or chocolate over boiled ham were automatically classified as "carbohydrate cravers".[9,10] Not surprisingly, "carbohydrate craving" was reported to characterize the vast majority of the obese population, including both men and women. Arguably, such a definition of "carbohydrate craving" is inadequate, and more attention should be paid to preferences for foods such as potatoes or bread.

In the present study, potatoes and bread were listed less frequently than either meat dishes or sweet desserts. Furthermore, these nonsweet carbohydrate sources tended to be listed largely by women and not by men. It might be argued on the basis of these data that there exists a population of female "carbohydrate cravers". However, preferences for carbohydrate sources are substantially less common than preferences for fat sources, and their contribution to human obesity syndromes has most likely been overstated.

## VI. CONCLUSIONS

Theories of macronutrients selection should recognize the central role of taste responsiveness and importance of hedonic response to food. People select and consume foods rather than macronutrients and individual food preferences are determined by a range of metabolic and behavioral variables. One promising central mechanism that may influence food selection involves endogenous opioid peptides. The opioid hypothesis links the central nervous system with sensory response to foods and should prove a productive area for further investigation.

## REFERENCES

1. The Surgeon General's Report on Nutrition and Health. DHHS (PHS) Publ. No. 88-50210, U.S. Government Printing Office, Washington, D.C., 1988.
2. Food and Nutrition Board, National Academy of Sciences. *Diet and Health.* National Academy Press, Washington D.C., 1989.
3. Schneeman, B., Fats in the diet: why and where?, *Food Technol.,* 40(10), 115, 1986.
5. Putler, D., and Frazad, E., Diet/health concerns about fat intake, *Food Rev.,* 1, 16, 1991.
6. Wurtman, J. J., Wurtman, R. J., Growdon, J. H., Henry, P., Lipscomb, A., and Zeisel, S., Carbohydrate craving in obese people: suppression by treatments affecting serotoninergic transmission, *Int. J. Eating Disord.,* 1, 2, 1981.
7. Wurtman, J., Wurtman, R., Mark, S., Tsay, R., Gilbert, W., and Growdon, J., d-Fenfluramine selectively suppresses carbohydrate snacking by obese subjects, *Int. J. Eating Disord.,* 4, 89, 1985.
8. Wurtman, J. J., The involvement of brain serotonin in excessive carbohydrate snacking by obese carbohydrate cravers, *J. Am. Dietetic Assoc.,* 84, 1004, 1984.
9. Lieberman, H. R., Wurtman, J. J., and Chew, B., Changes in mood after carbohydrate consumption among obese individuals, *Am. J. Clin. Nutr.,* 44, 772, 1986.

10. Heraief, E., Burckhardt, P., Wurtman, J. J., and Wurtman, R. J., Tryptophan administration may enhance weight loss by some moderately obese patients on a protein-sparing modified fast (PMSF) diet, *Int. J. Eating Disord.,* 4, 281, 1985.
11. Wurtman, J. J., and Wurtman, R. J., D-Fenfluramine selectively decreases carbohydrate but not protein intake in obese subjects, *Int. J. Obes.,* 8 (Suppl. 1), 79, 1984.
12. Romieu, I., Willett, W. C., Stampfer, M. J., Colditz, G. A., Sampson, L., Rosner, B., Hennekens, C. H., and Speizer, F. E., Energy intake and other determinants of relative weight, *Am. J. Clin. Nutr.,* 47, 406, 1988.
13. Dreon, D. M., Frey-Hewitt, B., Ellsworth, N., Williams, P. T., Terry, R. B., and Wood, P. D., Dietary fat: carbohydrate ratio and obesity in middle-aged men, *Am. J. Clin. Nutr.,* 47, 995, 1988.
14. Mela, D. J., and Sacchetti, D. A., Sensory preferences for fats: relationships with diet and body composition, *Am. J. Clin. Nutr.,* 53, 908, 1991.
15. Drewnowski, A., Taste and food preferences in human obesity. In: *Taste, Experience and Feeding,* E. D. Capaldi and T. L. Powley, Eds. American Psychological Association, Washington D.C., 1990.
16. Drewnowski, A., Brunzell, J., Sande, K., Iverius, P. H., and Greenwood, M. R. C., Sweet tooth reconsidered: taste responsiveness in human obesity, *Physiol. Behav.,* 35, 617, 1985.
17. Drewnowski, A., Pierce, B., and Halmi, K. A., Fat avoidance in eating disorders, *Appetite,* 10, 119, 1988.
18. Paykel, E. S., Mueller, P. S., and de la Vergne, P. M., Amitryptyline, weight gain and carbohydrate craving: a side effect, *Br. J. Psychiat.,* 123, 501, 1973.
19. Fernstrom, M. H., and Kupfer, D. J., Imipramine treatment and preference for sweets, *Appetite,* 10, 149, 1988.
20. Drewnowski, A., Krahn, D. D., Demitrack, M. A., Nairn, K., and Gosnell, B. A., Taste responses and preferences for sweet high-fat foods: evidence for opioid involvement, *Physiol. Behav.,* 51, 371, 1992.
21. Drewnowski, A., Fats and food texture: sensory and hedonic evaluations. In: *Food Texture,* H. R. Moskowitz, Ed. Marcel Dekker, New York, 1983, 629.
22. Drewnowski, A., Sensory preferences for fat and sugar in adolescence and adult life. In: *Nutrition and the Chemical Senses in Aging,* C. Murphy, W. S. Cain, and D. M. Hegsted, Eds. *Ann. N.Y. Acad. Sci.,* 561, 243, 1989.
23. Drewnowski, A., Fats and food texture: sensory and hedonic evaluations. In: *Food Texture,* H. R. Moskowitz, Ed. Marcel Dekker, New York, 1987, 251.
24. Wurtman, R. J., O'Rourke, D., and Wurtman, J. J., Nutrient imbalance in depressive disorders: possible brain mechanisms, In: *The Psychobiology of Human Eating Disorders,* L. H. Schneider, S. J. Cooper, and K. A. Halmi, Eds. *Ann. N.Y. Acad. Sci.,* 575, 75, 1989.
25. Rosenthal, N. E., Genhart, M., Jacobsen, F. M., Skwerer, R. G., and Wehr, T. A., Disturbance of appetite and weight regulation in seasonal affective disorder. In: *Human Obesity,* R. J. Wurtman and J. J. Wurtman, Eds., *Ann. N.Y. Acad. Sci.,* 499, 216, 1987.
26. Jenkins, D. J. A., Wolever, T. M. S., Taylor, R. H. et al., Glycemic index of foods: a physiological basis for carbohydrate exchange, *Am. J. Clin. Nutr.,* 34, 362, 1981.

27. Chiodo, J., and Latimer, P. R., Hunger perceptions and satiety responses among normal-weight bulimics and normals to a high-calorie, carbohydrate-rich food, *Psychol. Med.,* 16, 343, 1986.
28. Drewnowski, A., Changes in mood after carbohydrate consumption, *Am. J. Clin. Nutr.,* 46, 703, 1988.
29. Drewnowski, A., and Schwartz, M., Invisible fats: sensory assessment of sugar/fat mixtures, *Appetite,* 14, 203, 1990.
30. Anonymous. Could I be addicted to sweets?, *Lose Weight Naturally,* 4,10,1990.
31. Tomelleri, R., and Grunewald, K. K., Menstrual cycle and food cravings in young college women, *J. Am. Dietetic Assoc.,* 87, 311, 1987.
32. Drewnowski, A., Kurth, C., Holden-Wiltse, J., and Saari, J., Food preferences in human obesity: carbohydrates versus fats, *Appetite,* 18, 207, 1992.
33. Blass, E. M., Opioids, sugar and the inherent taste of sweet: broad motivational implications. In: *Sweetness,* J. Dobbing, Ed. Springer-Verlag, Berlin, 1987, 115.
34. Romsos, D. R., Gosnell, B. A., Morley, J. E., and Levine, A. S., Effects of kappa opiate agonists, cholecystokinin and bombesin on intake of diets varying in carbohydrate-to-fat ratio in rats, *J. Nutr.,* 117, 976, 1987.
35. Fantino, M., Hosotte, J., and Apfelbaum, M., An opioid antagonist naltrexone reduces preference for sucrose in humans, *Am. J. Physiol.,* 251: R9l, 1986.
36. Yeomans, M. R., Wright, P., Macleod, H. A., and Critchley, J. A. J. H., Effects of nalmefene on feeding in humans, *Psychopharmacology (Berlin),* 100, 426, 1990.
37. Volpicelli, J. R., Alterman, A. I., Hayashida, M., and O'Brien, C. P., Naltrexone in the treatment of alcohol dependence, *Arch. Gen. Psychiat.,* 49, 876, 1992.
38. Drewnowski, A., and Greenwood, M. R. C., Cream and sugar: human preferences for high-fat foods, *Physiol. Behav.,* 30, 629, 1983.
39. Drewnowski, A., Shrager, E. E., Lipsky, C., Stellar, E., and Greenwood, M. R. C., Sugar and fat: sensory and hedonic evaluations of liquid and solid foods, *Physiol. Behav.,* 45,177, 1989.
40. Meiselman, H. L., The role of sweetness in the food preferences of young adults. In: *Taste and Development: The Genesis of Sweet Preference,* J. M. Weiffenbach, Ed., DHEW Publ. No. (NIH) 77-1068, 1977.
41. Meiselman, H. L., and Waterman, D., Food preferences of enlisted personnel in the Armed Forces, *J. Am. Dietetic Assoc.,* 73, 621, 1978.
42. Gates, J. C., Huenemann, R. L., and Brand, R. J., Food choices of obese and non-obese persons, *J. Am. Dietetic Assoc.,* 76, 339, 1975.
43. Block, G., Dresser, C. M., Hartman, A. M., and Carroll, M. D., Nutrient sources in the American diet: quantitative data from the NHANES II survey, *Am. J. Epidemiol.,* 122, 27, 1985.

# 11 Fat Substitutes and Regulation of Food Intake in Rats

**Ruth B. S. Harris**

## I. INTRODUCTION

Fat-free food products have been developed by the food industry in response to the increase in consumer awareness of the potential health benefits of reducing fat intake[1] and to mandates from health professional organizations to provide an increased number of low-fat or reduced fat alternative food choices.[2,3] Lyle et al.[4] calculated that if seven categories of fat-free foods totally replaced the use of their full fat counterparts then median fat intake of the United States population would fall from approximately 36 to 30% of dietary energy. Several studies have shown that when the fat content of a meal is covertly replaced with a fat substitute subjects compensate for the decrease in energy intake but not for the reduction in fat intake, resulting in a lower total 24-h fat intake.[5,6]

Experiments using animal models allow investigation of the physiological impact of using extreme levels of fat replacement, which could not be achieved consistently in a clinical trial, and permit measurements that may not be possible with human subjects. Several studies have been completed to examine the effects of fat replacement on energy balance, body composition, lipid metabolism, and nutrient partitioning in rats.

## II. EXTREME CHANGES IN FAT INTAKE

Although it has been established that essential fatty acids are required to support normal growth,[7,8] there is little information available concerning the minimum level of nonessential dietary fat required in an otherwise

0-8493-4466-2/94/$0.00+$.50

nutritionally complete diet. Forbes et al.[9] reported that there was little difference in growth of rats fed diets containing 5, 10, or 30% corn oil although both nitrogen and fat gains were depressed by a diet containing only 2% oil. Noncaloric fat substitutes provide an opportunity to examine the effects of palatable, nutritionally complete, very low-fat diets on various physiological functions.

### A. Growing Animals

Low-fat diets in which fat had been replaced with a carbohydrate-based fat mimetic were used to determine the impact of removing nonessential dietary fat on growth in young rats.[10] Male Sprague-Dawley rats (45 g) were housed two per cage with food and water freely available. Four weight matched groups were each fed one of the four diets described in Table 1 for 27 days. In the control diet approximately 17% of energy was derived from fat. The high-fat diet supplied approximately 36% of energy as fat. Two low-fat diets were made by replacing the fat in the control and the high-fat diets with a fat mimetic. Essential fatty acids supplied the only lipid in the low-fat diets, providing approximately 4% of energy.

Animals fed high or low-fat diets adjusted food intake so that there were no differences in digestible energy intakes of the four groups (Table 2), however, by the end of the experiment rats fed the low-fat diets were approximately 20 g heavier than those fed either the 17 or 36% kcal fat diets. Daily body weights are shown in Figure 1. Carcass composition, shown in Table 2, indicated that the greater weight gain in these rats was totally accounted for by an increase in lean body mass. There were no significant differences in total body fat content or epididymal fat pad weights of the four groups. Replacement of nonessential fat with a noncaloric mimetic raised the proportion of dietary energy supplied by protein and carbohydrate and it is possible that an increased protein-calorie ratio was responsible for the improved growth of lean tissue in animals fed low-fat diets.

There was no indication that the rats adjusted food intake to achieve a constant fat intake, suggesting that there was no specific appetite for fat. The precise compensation for a reduction in dietary energy concentration demonstrated that nutritionally complete, very low-fat diets do not reduce essential nutrient intake of young animals as long as the food supply is not restricted.

### B. Mature Animals

A second study was conducted to characterize physiological responses made by mature rats to diets in which part, or all, nonessential fat was replaced with a substitute.[11] Adult virgin female rats that had reached a relatively stable weight were used so that changes in body weight would be largely attributable to changes in fat content and would not be complicated by growth.

**TABLE 1**
**Composition of Control, High-Fat, and Very Low-Fat Diets (g/kg) Offered to Growing Rats for 28 Days**

| | Control | Low-fat I | High-fat | Low-fat II |
|---|---|---|---|---|
| Casein | 200 | 200 | 200 | 200 |
| Corn oil | 67 | — | 160 | — |
| Coconut oil | 13 | — | 30 | — |
| Fat mimetic[a] | — | 62 | — | 172 |
| Linoleic acid | — | 18 | — | 18 |
| Vitamin mix[b] | 10 | 10 | 10 | 10 |
| Mineral mix[b] | 34 | 34 | 34 | 34 |
| Alphacel | 40 | 40 | 40 | 40 |
| Sucrose | 316 | 316 | 261 | 261 |
| Starch | 316 | 316 | 261 | 261 |
| DL-Methionine | 4 | 4 | 4 | 4 |
| Digestible energy[c] (kcal/g) | 4.46 | 3.71 | 5.07 | 3.78 |
| Energy from protein %kcal | 18.9 | 21.7 | 16.7 | 24.7 |

[a] The composition of the fat mimetic was 5.9% cellulose, 0.3% xanthan, and 93.8% water.

[b] The compositions of mineral and vitamin mixes have been described in detail elsewhere.[10]

[c] Digestible energy of the diets was determined by bomb calorimetery of diet and feces.

Female Sprague-Dawley rats, weighing approximately 220 g, were divided into five groups matched for average body weight. Each group was fed one of five diets for 64 days. The control (21% kcal fat) diet contained 10%, by weight, corn oil. A low-fat (2% kcal fat) diet was made by replacing the oil in the control diet with a protein-based fat substitute supplemented with linoleic acid to prevent fatty acid deficiency. The high-fat (63% kcal fat) diet contained 10% corn oil and 30% Crisco (Procter & Gamble, Cincinnati, OH), by weight. In two other diets, half or all of the Crisco was replaced with the substitute, resulting in diets that provided 51 and 30% kcal from fat. Replacement of Crisco with the fat substitute increased the proportion of dietary energy supplied by protein from 14% in the 63% kcal fat diet to 28% in the 30% kcal fat diet. Food was available *ad libitum* and replaced daily.

Final body weights of the rats and food and energy intakes recorded during the last 14 days of the experiment are shown in Table 3. Rats offered the 63%

**TABLE 2**
**Food Intake and Body Composition of Growing Rats Fed Very Low-Fat Diets[a]**

| | Control | Low-fat I | High-fat | Low-fat II |
|---|---|---|---|---|
| Food intake (g/2 rats/day) | 28.4 ± 0.8[a] | 33.3 ± 0.3[b] | 25.1 ± 0.5[c] | 35.0 ± 0.7[d] |
| Energy intake (kcal/2 rats/day) | 127 ± 4 | 124 ± 1 | 127 ± 3 | 132 ± 3 |
| Carcass weight (g) | 214 ± 3[a] | 236 ± 3[b] | 211 ± 5[a] | 228 ± 3[b] |
| Fat (g) | 14 ± 0.8 | 16 ± 0.8 | 14 ± 0.4 | 14 ± 0.8 |
| Protein (g) | 51 ± 0.4[a] | 54 ± 0.8[b] | 51 ± 1.2[a] | 54 ± 0.8[b] |
| Water (g) | 136 ± 4[a] | 157 ± 3[b] | 139 ± 3[a] | 152 ± 2[b] |
| Epididymal fat (g) | 2.1 ± 0.1 | 2.0 ± 0.1 | 2.0 ± 0.1 | 2.0 ± 0.1 |

[a] Data are means ± SEM for groups of 10 male Sprague-Dawley rats fed either a control 17% kcal fat diet, a high-fat 36% kcal fat diet, or low-fat diets in which all fat except essential fatty acids had been replaced with a fat mimetic. Values for a given parameter that do not share a common superscript are significantly different at $p < 0.05$, determined by one-way analysis of variance and calculation of least significant difference.

kcal fat diet had lower food intakes but significantly higher energy intakes than the control rats. Rats given the 30% kcal fat diet consumed approximately 140% as much food as controls so that, although the diet was less energetically dense than the control diet, they still had a higher energy intake than controls. Rats receiving the 51% kcal fat had a food intake that was higher than that of controls and an energy intake that was the same as that of rats fed the 63% kcal fat diet. By the end of the experiment weight gain reflected energy intake, in that the 63 and 51% kcal fat rats were significantly heavier than the 30% kcal fat rats, which were heavier than controls. All of the weight differences between groups were accounted for by carcass fat content so that nonsignificant differences in body weight were significant when attributed to fat content (Table 3). There were no differences in carcass protein content.

Failure to accurately compensate for increased energy concentration in the high-fat diets was consistent with previous reports that rats become obese when given a high-fat diet.[12] The rats reduced food intake compared with controls but not sufficiently to prevent the development of obesity. Although energy intakes of rats fed the 51% kcal fat diet were the same as those of rats fed the 63% kcal fat diet their body fat content was significantly less. These data are consistent with observations that rats,[3] mice,[14] and humans[15] are less efficient at utilizing energy from dietary carbohydrate

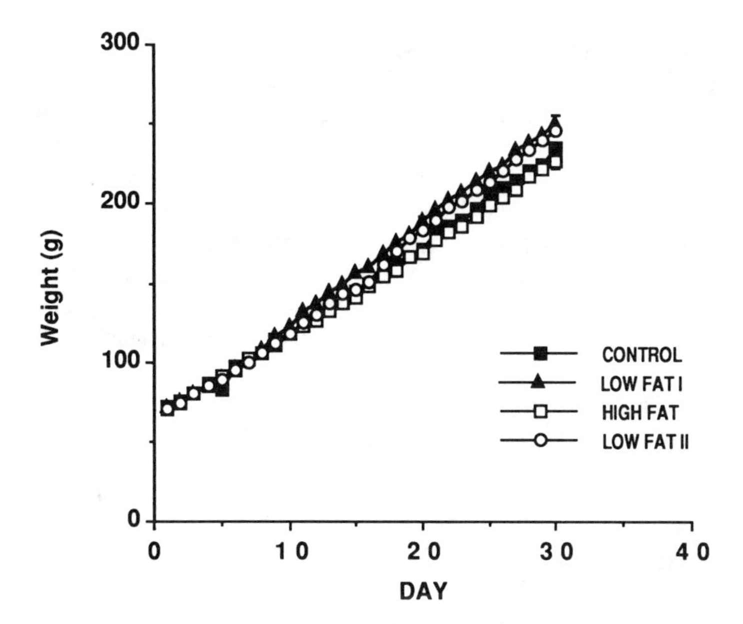


**FIGURE 1.** Mean daily body weights of young male Sprague-Dawley rats given free access to diets containing different amounts of fat.

## TABLE 3
## Food Intake, Energy Intake, Body Composition, and Serum Glucose and Insulin of Mature Rats Offered Either a Very Low-Fat or Very High-Fat Diets[a]

| | 2% kcal fat | 21% kcal fat | 30% kcal fat | 51% kcal fat | 63% kcal fat |
|---|---|---|---|---|---|
| Food intake (g/14 d) | 149 ± 3[b] | 176 ± 3[c] | 210 ± 5[d] | 163 ± 5[bc] | 129 ± 3[a] |
| Energy intake (kcal/14 d) | 627 ± 13[ab] | 598 ± 12[a] | 673 ± 15[bc] | 725 ± 22[cd] | 734 ± 17[d] |
| Carcass measures | | | | | |
| Weight (g) | 213 ± 4[a] | 219 ± 2[a] | 231 ± 2[b] | 246 ± 5[c] | 252 ± 6[c] |
| Fat (g) | 17.8 ± 0.8[a] | 18.3 ± 0.7[a] | 26.4 ± 1.0[b] | 34.6 ± 1.3[c] | 42.8 ± 4.5[d] |
| Protein (g) | 44.9 ± 2.3 | 45.5 ± 2.0 | 48.0 ± 1.6 | 49.5 ± 1.1 | 49.2 ± 1.2 |
| Serum measures | | | | | |
| Glucose (mmol/L) | 5.6 ± 0.2 | 6.0 ± 0.1 | 6.0 ± 0.2 | 6.2 ± 0.2 | 5.9 ± 0.3 |
| Insulin (pmol/L) | 194 ± 14[a] | 237 ± 7[a] | 201 ± 7[a] | 222 ± 7[a] | 352 ± 43[b] |

[a] Data are means ± SEM for groups of 10 rats. Values for a given parameter that do not share a common superscript are significantly different at $p < 0.05$.

than from dietary fat. As the occurrence of obesity has been associated with consumption of a high-fat diet,[16] fat-free foods that retain the physical and sensory properties of high-fat foods have the potential to reduce the risk for development of obesity.

In this experiment there were no differences in energy intakes of control (21% kcal fat fed) and 2% kcal fat fed rats. Thus replacement of relatively low levels of nonessential fat had no effect on body weight or body composition. In a previously reported study, when rats were offered diets in which 15% fat was replaced with the totally nondigestible fat substitute sucrose polyester they increased food intake to compensate for the reduction in dietary energy concentration.[17] Addition of nonabsorbable sucrose polyester to a diet may inhibit absorption of fat-soluble nutrients, including cholesterol[18] and Vitamin A.[17] In this study the fat substitute was protein-based and fully digestible, therefore, although no measurements were made to assess absorption of fat-soluble nutrients, it seems unlikely that their absorption would be inhibited.

At the end of this experiment rats receiving the 63% kcal fat diet were hyperinsulinemic whereas the 51% kcal fat fed animals were not (Table 3), suggesting that even low levels of fat replacement may have a beneficial effect on insulin sensitivity and responsiveness. To confirm this observation rats were fed a 21, a 63, or a 2% kcal fat diet for 50 days at the end of which epididymal adipocyte insulin responsiveness was measured.[19] Although muscle accounts for the majority of glucose utilization *in vivo,* adipocytes are considered a good insulin-responsive model for muscle.[20] Total lipid synthesis, measured by *in vitro* incorporation of radiolabeled glucose into triglyceride fatty acids, indicated that adipocytes from rats fed the high-fat diet were insulin resistant whereas adipocytes from animals fed the control and low-fat diet appeared to be equally sensitive to insulin (Figure 2). Therefore, although very high-fat diets caused insulin insensitivity, reduction of dietary fat to very low levels had no effect on insulin responsiveness beyond that achieved with a 20% kcal fat diet.

The studies described above demonstrate that rats can adapt to very low-fat diets. In young rats normal growth is maintained as long as essential fatty acids are present in the diet and energy intake is not restricted. Low-fat diets may even promote deposition of lean tissue if the protein-calorie ratio of the diet is increased compared with a high-fat diet. Mature rats compensate for the reduced energy density of very low-fat diets so that there is no effect on energy intake or body composition. Rats fed very high-fat diets have an increased energy intake, which leads to the development of obesity and insulin resistance. The degree of obesity appeared to be proportional to the fat content of the diet and insulin resistance was moderated when only a portion of the fat was replaced. Comparison of responses of rats fed high-fat and low-fat diets suggested that there was a threshold level for dietary

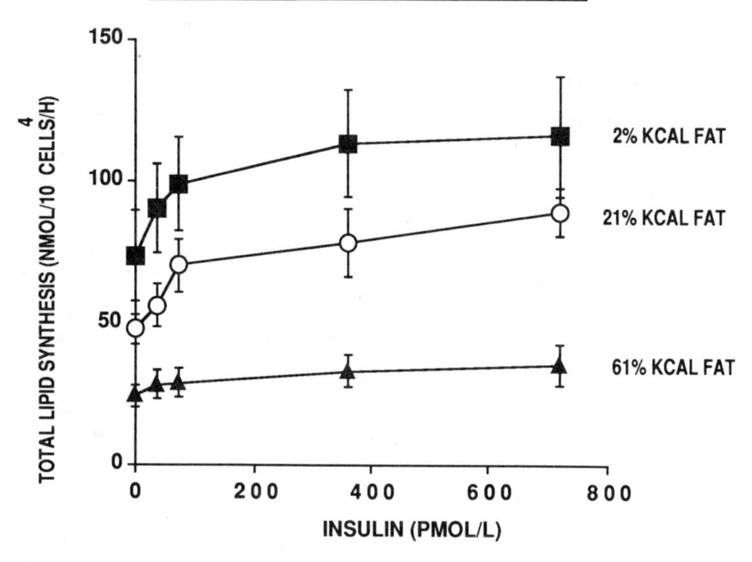


**FIGURE 2.** Adipocyte total lipid synthesis measured in inguinal cells obtained from female Sprague-Dawley rats that had been fed diets containing different levels of fat for 30 days. Lipid synthesis was measured *in vitro* by incorporation of [U-$^{14}$C] glucose in triglyceride fatty acids.[19]

fat content that stimulates overfeeding and development of obesity in rats. Below this threshold the animals regulated energy balance to maintain a constant body composition.

## III. MODERATE CHANGES IN FAT INTAKE

Health professionals are recommending that individuals reduce their fat intake to 30%, or less, of dietary energy.[2,3] Lyle et al.[4] reported that use of currently available fat-free processed foods could potentially facilitate achievement of this goal. Therefore, several animal studies were completed to compare the responses of rats fed diets containing either 30 or 40% of calories from fat.

### A. Mature Animals

In animals it has been shown that both the type and level of dietary fatty acid influences insulin function in adipose tissue.[21,22] Insulin resistance caused by diets containing high levels of fat or a high proportion of saturated fat has been attributed to a reduction in the number of glucose transporters in the intracellular pool.[23,24] It has been suggested that obesity may lead to the development of insulin insensitivity and unresponsiveness independent of the direct effect of dietary fat on insulin sensitivity.[25] Insulin resistance in human obesity has been associated with both binding and postbinding defects in cells[26] possibly initiated by chronic exposure of tissue to high levels of insulin.[27,28]

An experiment[29] was designed to determine whether a diet containing 40% of energy as fat caused insulin insensitivity or resistance in rats and, if so, whether reduction of dietary fat to 30% of energy would correct the response. Three diets were used in this study, a high-fat diet containing 40% energy as fat, a control diet in which some fat was replaced with starch and sucrose to reduce dietary fat to 30% of energy, and a mimetic diet that also contained 30% kcal fat but the fat had been replaced with a carbohydrate-based fat mimetic. Casein supplied 16% calories in all three diets. The ratio of saturated to polyunsaturated to monounsaturated fatty acids was kept constant by maintaining the ratio of corn oil to coconut oil.

Mature (250 g) female Sprague-Dawley rats were fed either the high-fat diet or the control 30% kcal fat diet for 10 weeks. Glucose tolerance was measured in six rats from each dietary group and then some animals that had been fed the 40% kcal fat diet were switched to either the control 30% kcal fat diet (HF/C) or were switched to the mimetic 30% kcal fat diet (HF/M). Three days later glucose tolerance was measured. The experimental design is illustrated in Figure 3.

The results of the two *in vivo* glucose tolerance measurements are shown in Figures 4 and 5, respectively. When the control and high-fat rats were compared at the end of the 10-week feeding period there was a significant effect of diet on serum insulin response to the glucose challenge. Rats fed the high-fat diet demonstrated a greater insulin release at the initiation of the challenge and basal insulin concentrations appeared to be elevated. Hyperinsulinemia in the presence of normal plasma glucose concentrations indicated insulin insensitivity in these animals. In the second glucose tolerance test, 3 days after the diet switch, there was also a significant effect of diet on insulin response. Rats fed the high-fat diet were insulin insensitive, giving an exaggerated insulin response to the glucose challenge. However, 3 days on a 30% kcal fat diet had caused a reversal of the insulin insensitivity induced by the 40% kcal fat diet. Insulin response and basal insulin concentration measured in HF/C rats were no different from those of controls. In HF/M rats basal insulin concentrations were the same as those of controls and the insulin response to the glucose challenge was only slightly exaggerated. These measurements indicate that impaired glucose tolerance responds very rapidly to a reduction in dietary fat intake, independent of the means used to replace

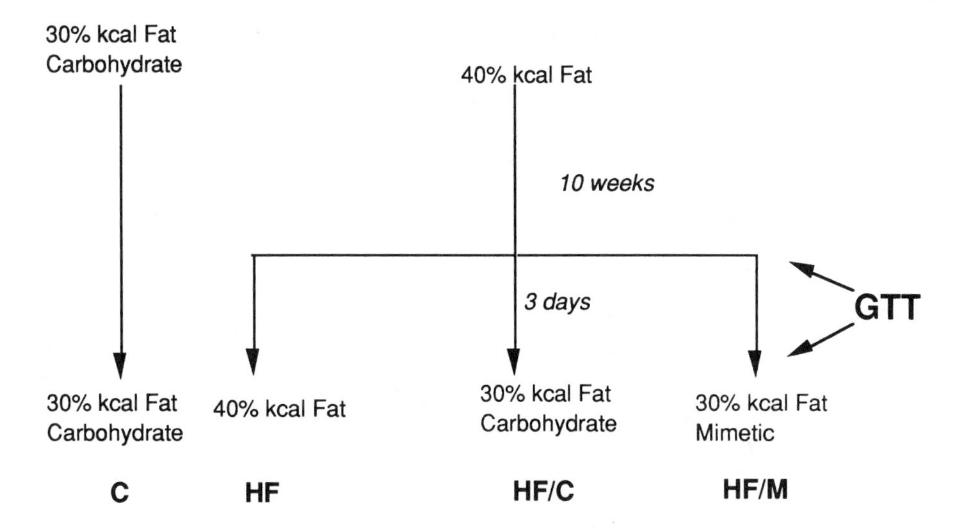


**FIGURE 3.** Experimental design of a study intended to measure the effects of feeding diets containing 40 or 30% of energy as fat on *in vivo* glucose tolerance of rats. *In vivo* glucose tolerance was measured on control (C) (HF) and high-fat-fed rats after 10 weeks and on C, HF, HF/C, and HF/M fed rats 3 days after diets were switched.[29]

the fat, and suggests that insulin insensitivity induced by a high-fat diet is directly related to the level of fat in the diet, rather than occurring as a secondary response to increased body fat content[25] or enlargement of adipocytes.[30]

In this study rats fed a 40% kcal fat diet had higher energy intakes (583 vs. 533 kcal/10 days) and were fatter (14 vs. 10% carcass fat) than those fed the 30% kcal fat diet, implying that a relatively small increase in dietary fat content from 30 to 40% of energy was sufficient to cause hyperphagia. The differences in body composition were confirmed in another study in which rats were offered diets containing different ratios of macronutrients. Figure 6 shows that after 65 days rats fed a diet containing 40% of energy as fat weighed significantly more than those fed diets containing 30% energy as fat, irrespective of the ratios of protein or carbohydrate to fat in those diets. Carcass analysis indicated that 70% of the difference in weight was due to an increase in body fat content.

## B. Growing Animals

Health professionals have made recommendations for children over 2 years of age that are similar to those for adults: to reduce fat intake to approximately 30% of energy intake and to consume a varied balanced

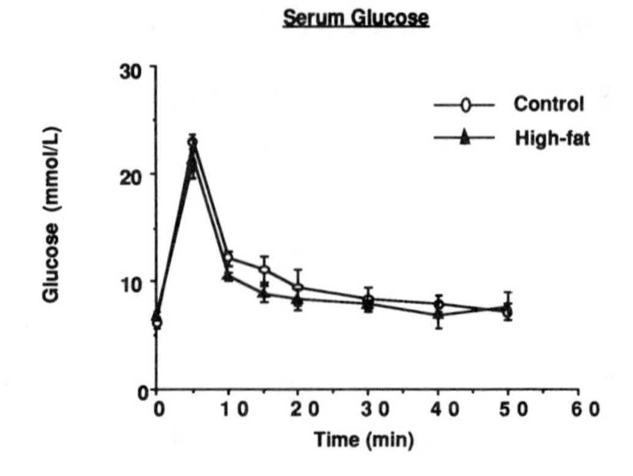


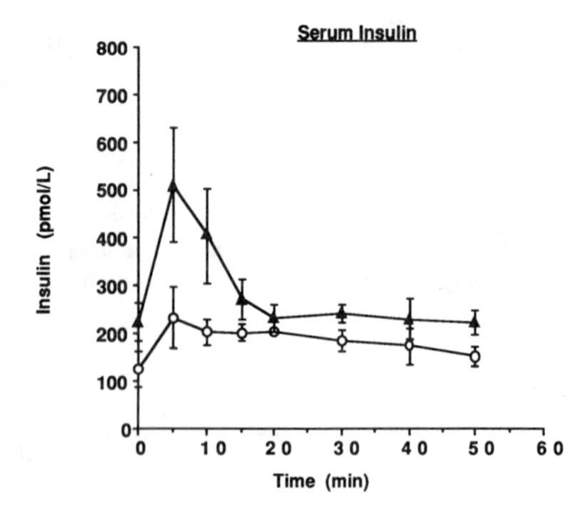


**FIGURE 4.** *In vivo* glucose tolerance measured in five anesthetized rats from each of the high-fat and control groups of rats at the end of the 10-week feeding period. Values are means ± SEM. Each rat was given 1 mg/kg glucose intravenously and blood samples were taken via a jugular cannula at 0, 5, 10, 15, 20, 30, 40, or 50 min after injection. There was a significant effect of diet on serum insulin concentration ($p < 0.001$, $LSD_{0.05}$ 22.1).

diet,[31,32] however, there is some hesitation to recommend that children consume fat-modified foods as fat is an energy-dense ingredient that carries micronutrients essential for normal growth and development. Simultaneously there is concern that the occurrence and severity of adolescent obesity is increasing[33] possibly linked to an increased amount of time spent watching television[34] and an increased consumption of high-fat snack foods.[35] It is difficult to treat adolescent obesity by traditional methods as food restriction may inhibit longitudinal growth[36] and the success of behavior modification varies between individuals[37] being most successful when parents and children are involved in the program.[38]

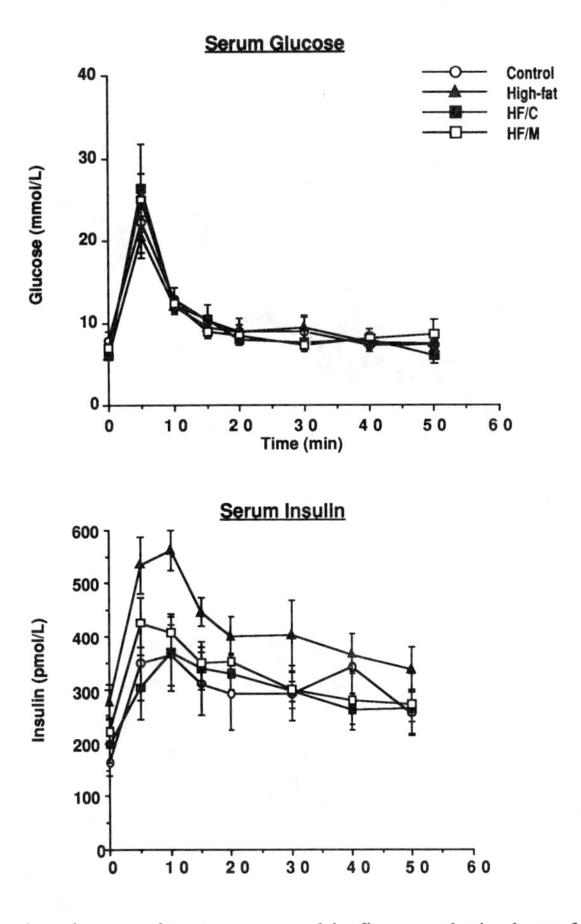


**FIGURE 5.** *In vivo* glucose tolerance measured in five anesthetized rats from each of the high-fat, control, HF/C, and HF/M groups 3 days after the diet was switched. Values are means ± SEM. Each rat was given 1 mg/kg glucose intravenously and blood samples were taken by jugular cannula at 0, 5, 10, 15, 20, 30, 40, and 50 min after injection. There was a significant effect of diet on serum insulin concentration ($p < 0.001$, $LSD_{0.05}$ 21.4).

The experiment described at the beginning of this chapter demonstrated that young rats are able to maintain a normal rate of growth on diets that contain very low concentrations of fat.[10] The objective of the next experiment was to determine whether replacement of full fat foods with low-fat or fat-free counterparts would impact energy intake and body composition in growing rats. Cafeteria diets have typically been used to induce obesity in rats[39] and were considered an appropriate model for dietary induced obesity.

Young (90 g) male Sprague-Dawley rats, in the rapid stage of growth, were fed either a 30% kcal fat diet or the diet plus either a low-fat or a

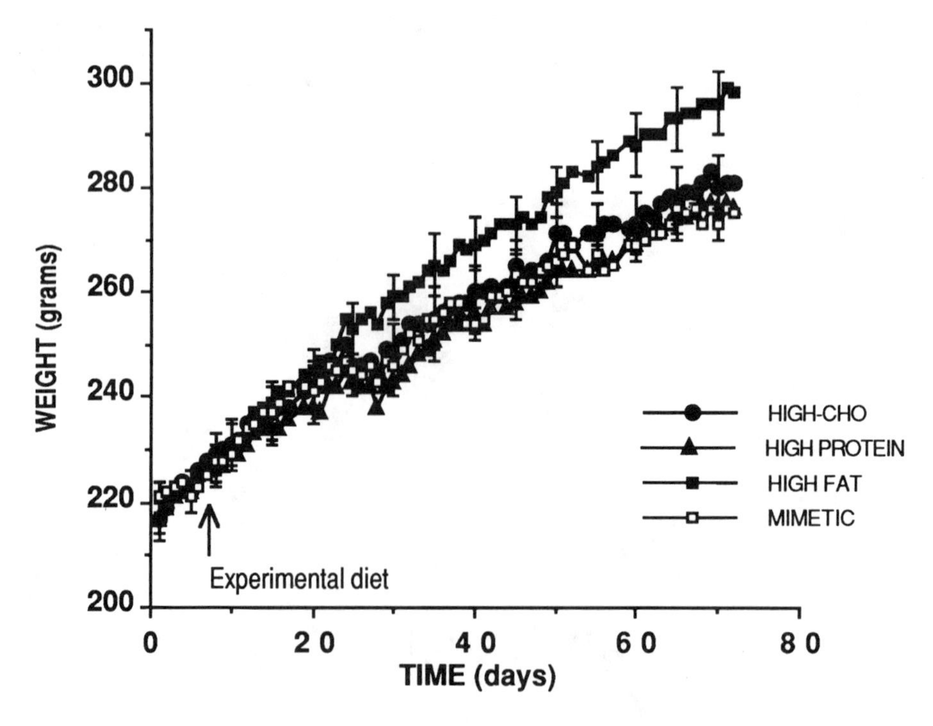


**FIGURE 6.** Mean daily body weights for groups of 10 female Sprague-Dawley rats fed diets containing either 40 or 30% of energy as fat. The ratio of macronutrients in each of the 30% kcal fat diets was varied so that the high-CHO diet contained 16% of energy as protein and 54% as carbohydrate. The high protein diet contained 26% of energy as protein and 44% as carbohydrate. The mimetic diet was made by replacing some of the fat in the 40% kcal fat diet with a carbohydrate-based fat mimetic. This diet contained 19% of energy as protein and 51% as carbohydrate. The 40% kcal fat diet contained 16% of energy as protein and 43% as carbohydrate.

high-fat cafeteria food each day for 38 days. The high-fat cafeteria foods used were salad dressing, chocolate, chocolate chip cookies, potato chips, and bologna. The low-fat foods were fat-free salad dressing, raisins, marshmallows, fat-free oatmeal raisin cookies, and 98% fat-free turkey. As the rats received only one cafeteria food each day it was possible to measure intake of both diet and cafeteria foods during the experimental period.

There was no effect of diet on rate of weight gain or on final body weight of the rats. Offering either low-fat or high-fat cafeteria foods decreased the intake of purified diet. When total food intake was considered animals given cafeteria foods ate more than those offered only diet and rats offered low-fat foods ate more than those offered high-fat foods. Although a greater

**TABLE 4**
**Food and Energy Intakes and Body Composition of Young Rats Fed Either a 30% kcal Fat Diet or Diet Plus Cafeteria Foods for 38 Days[a]**

| | Control | Low-fat cafeteria | High-fat cafeteria |
|---|---|---|---|
| Diet consumption (g/38 d) | 693 ± 6[a] | 501 ± 10[b] | 499 ± 19[b] |
| Total food intake (g/38 d) | 693 ± 6[a] | 968 ± 13[b] | 799 ± 26[c] |
| Total energy intake (kcal/38 d) | 3096 ± 20[a] | 3202 ± 42[b] | 3721 ± 121[c] |
| Carcass measures | | | |
| Weight (g) | 354 ± 4 | 348 ± 5 | 356 ± 7 |
| Fat (g) | 27.7 ± 2.4[a] | 23.0 ± 1.6[b] | 29.6 ± 2.0[a] |
| Protein (g) | 90.5 ± 1.5 | 90.5 ± 1.5 | 91.4 ± 2.0 |

[a] Data are means ± SEM for groups of seven or eight rats. Values for a given parameter that do not share a common superscript are significantly different at $p < 0.05$, determined by one-way analysis of variance and calculation of least significant difference.

quantity of low-fat cafeteria foods was consumed, more energy was obtained from the high-fat cafeteria foods (Table 4). The proportion of dietary energy obtained from fat, protein and carbohydrate as a percent of total energy intake is shown in Figure 7. Low-fat cafeteria foods resulted in a decrease in the percentage of energy obtained from fat, to about 24%, did not change the percent energy intake from protein and increased percent energy from carbohydrate. High-fat cafeteria foods increased the percent energy obtained from fat, to about 43%, and decreased the amount of energy consumed as either protein or carbohydrate.

Dietary treatment had no effect on any carcass parameter measured except carcass fat content. This was the same in control and high-fat cafeteria rats but was reduced in low-fat cafeteria rats (Table 4). The consistent rate of growth between treatment groups also indicated that although the high-fat cafeteria foods reduced the proportion of energy obtained from protein, all of the rats consumed an adequate amount of protein and had an appropriate protein:calorie ratio to support optimal growth.

Low-fat foods reduced both energy intake and the proportion of dietary energy obtained from fat compared with high-fat foods. These responses to

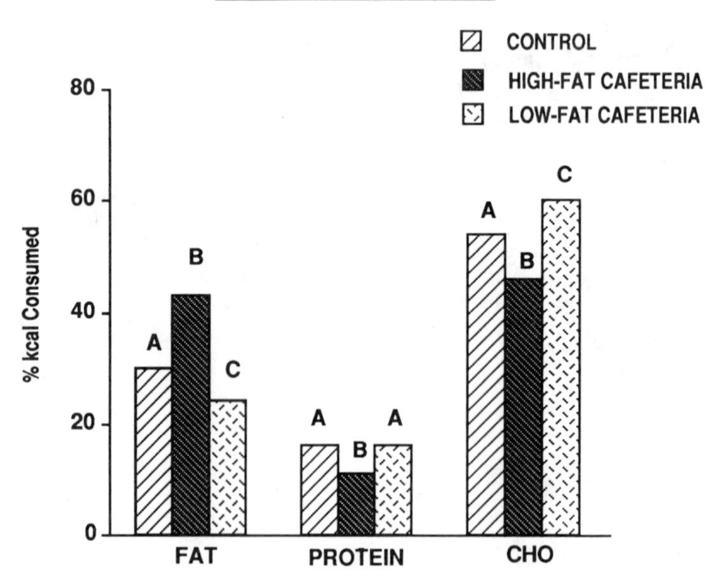


**FIGURE 7.** Macronutrient intake of young male Sprague-Dawley rats offered either a 30% kcal fat diet or diet plus either a high-fat or a low-fat cafeteria food each day. Values are expressed as percent of total energy consumed during the experiment.

low-fat foods may be beneficial, especially in a situation in which there is a risk of development of obesity. Flatt[14] hypothesized that food intake is controlled to maintain nutrient balance. To maintain nutrient balance with a high-fat diet fatty acid oxidation must be stimulated and this is achieved by increasing body fat content and decreasing glycogen stores. Recent studies investigating the responses of adult human subjects to reduced fat diets have also demonstrated a reduction in body weight when the proportion of dietary energy obtained from fat was decreased.[15,40,41] If low-fat foods reduce both total energy intake and percent energy obtained from fat, compared with high-fat foods, there should be beneficial effects on both body weight and composition due to shifts in both energy balance and nutrient partitioning.

These studies examining the responses of rats to moderate changes in fat intake show that increasing dietary fat content from 30 to 40% of dietary energy can induce hyperphagia, obesity, and insulin resistance. The insulin resistance may be a primary response to dietary fat content, rather than secondary to an increase in body fat content. Growing animals offered low-fat snack foods had a lower energy intake and a reduced body fat content compared with animals receiving high-fat snack foods, suggesting that diets that include low-fat or fat-free foods should be evaluated as a possible means of reducing risk for obesity in adolescents.

## IV. CONCLUSIONS

Animal studies examining responses made to extreme and moderate changes in dietary fat content indicate that the beneficial effects of reducing dietary fat include a lower voluntary energy intake, a reduced body fat content, and improved insulin sensitivity. The responses occur independently of the means used to reduce fat content. There were no unique responses to diets containing fat mimetics and lowering the fat content of the diet did not appear to have any adverse effects on growth. These results support the suggestion that fat-free foods may be used as a convenient means of reducing the fat intake of the general population.[42]

## REFERENCES


1. Food Marketing Institute, Nutrition. In: *Trends: Consumer Attitudes and the Supermarket,* Louis Harris & Associates Inc., Washington, D.C., 1990, chap. 5.
2. National Research Council, *Diet and Health: Implications for Reducing Chronic Disease Risk,* National Academy of Science Press, Washington, D.C., 1989.
3. U.S. Department of Health and Human Services, *Promoting Health/Preventing Disease: Year 2000 Objectives for the Nation,* Public Health Service, Washington, D.C., 1989.
4. Lyle, B. J., McMahon, K. E., and Kreutler, P. A., Assessing the potential dietary impact of replacing dietary fat with other macronutrients, *J. Nutr.,* 122, 211, 1992.
5. Rolls, B. J., Dietary fat and regulation of food intake in adults, *Int. J. Obes.,* 15, MS16, 1991.
6. Birch, L., and Johnson, S. L., Appetite control in children, This volume.
7. Burr, G. O., and Burr, M. M., A new deficiency disease produced by the rigid exclusion of fat from the diet, *J. Biol. Chem.,* 82, 345, 1929.
8. Holman, R. J., The ratio of trienoic:tetraenoic acids in tissue lipids as a measure of fatty acid requirement, *J. Nutr.,* 70, 405, 1960.
9. Forbes, E. B., Swift, R. W., Elliot, R. F., and James, W. H., Relation of fat to economy of food utilization I. By the growing albino rat, *J. Nutr.,* 31, 203, 1946.
10. Harris, R. B. S., Growth measurements in Sprague-Dawley rats fed diets of very low-fat concentration, *J. Nutr.,* 121, 1075, 1991.
11. Harris, R. B. S., and Jones, W. K., Physiological response of mature rats to replacement of dietary fat with a fat substitute, *J. Nutr.,* 121, 1109, 1991.
12. Schemmel, R., Mickelson, O., and Motawi, K., Conversion of dietary to body energy in rats as affected by strain, sex and ration, *J. Nutr.,* 102, 1187, 1972.
13. Donato, K., and Hegsted, D. M., Efficiency of utilization of various sources of energy for growth, *Proc. Natl. Acad. Sci. U.S.A.,* 82, 4866, 1985.
14. Flatt, J. P., Dietary fat, carbohydrate balance, and weight maintenance: effects of exercise, *Am. J. Clin. Nutr.,* 45, 296, 1987.

15. Prewitt, T. E., Schmeisser, D., Bowen, P. E., Aye, P., Dolecek, T. A., Langenberg, P., Cole, T., and Brace, L., Changes in body weight, body composition, and energy intake in women fed high- and low-fat diets, *Am. J. Clin. Nutr.*, 54, 304, 1991.
16. Danforth, E., Diet and obesity, *Am. J. Clin. Nutr.*, 41, 1132, 1985.
17. Mattson, F. H., Hollenbach, E. J., and Kuehlthau, C., The effect of a non-absorbable fat, sucrose polyester, on the metabolism of Vitamin A by the rat, *J. Nutr.*, 109, 1688, 1979.
18. Jandacek, R. J., Mattso, F. H., McNeely, S., Gallon, L., Yunker, R., and Glueck, C. J., Effect of sucrose polyester on fecal steroid excretion by 24 normal men, *Am. J. Clin. Nutr.*, 33, 251, 1980.
19. Harris, R. B. S., Adipocyte insulin responsiveness in female Sprague-Dawley rats fed a high-fat or a low-fat diet containing a carbohydrate fat mimetic, *J. Nutr.*, 122, 1802, 1992.
20. Simpson, I. A., and Cushman, S. W., Hormonal regulation of mammalian glucose transport, *Annu. Rev. Biochem.*, 55, 1059, 1986.
21. van Amelsvoort, J. M. M., van der Beek, A., and Stam, J. J., Dietary influence on the insulin function in the epididymal fat cell of the Wistar rat. III. Effect of the ratio carbohydrate to fat, *Ann. Nutr. Metab.*, 32, 160, 1988.
22. van Amelsvoort, J. M. M., van der Beek, A., Stam, J. J., and Houtsmuller, U. M. T., Dietary influence on the insulin function in the epididymal fat cell of the Wistar rat. I. Effect of type of fat, *Ann. Nutr. Metab.*, 32, 138, 1988.
23. Hissin, P. J., Karnelli, E., Simpson, I. A., Salans, L. B., and Cushman, S. W., A possible mechanism of insulin resistance in the rat adipose cell with high-fat/low-carbohydrate feeding. Depletion of intracellular glucose transport systems, *Diabetes*, 31, 589, 1982.
24. Lee, H-C. C., and Dupont, J., Effects of dietary fatty acids on the activity of glucose transport in adipocytes, *J. Nutr. Biochem.*, 2, 38, 1991.
25. Hanson, B. C., Jen, K-L. C., and Schwartz, J., Changes in insulin responses and binding in adipocytes from monkeys with obesity progressing towards diabetes, *Int. J. Obes.*, 12, 433, 1987.
26. Kolterman, O. G., Insel, J., and Saekow, M., Mechanisms of insulin resistance in human obesity. Evidence for receptor and post-receptor defects, *J. Clin. Invest.*, 65, 1272, 1980.
27. Marangou, A. G., Weber, K. M., Boston, R. C., Aitken, P. M., Heggie, J. C. P., Kirsner, R. L. G., Best, J. D., and Alford, F. P., Metabolic consequences of prolonged hyperinsulinemia in humans. Evidence for induction of insulin insensitivity, *Diabetes*, 35, 1383, 1986.
28. Bonadonna, R. C., Groop, L., Kraemer, N., Ferrannini, E., Del Pratto, S., and DeFronzo, R. A., Obesity and insulin resistance in humans: a dose response study, *Metabolism*, 39, 452, 1990.
29. Harris, R. B. S., and Kor, H., Insulin insensitivity is rapidly reversed in rats by reducing dietary fat from 40% to 30% of energy, *J. Nutr.*, 122, 1811, 1992.
30. Olefsky, J. M., Mechanisms of decreased insulin responsiveness of large adipocytes, *Endocrinology*, 100, 1169, 1977.
31. American Academy of Pediatrics Committee on Nutrition. Prudent life-style for children: dietary fat and cholesterol, *Pediatrics*, 78, 521, 1986.

32. Weidman, W., Kwiterovich, P., Jesse, M. J., and Nugent, E., AHA Committee Report. Diet in the healthy child, *Circulation,* 67, 1411A, 1984.
33. Gortmarker, S. L., Dietz, W. H., Sobol, A. M., and Wehler, C. A., Increasing pediatric obesity in the United States, *Am. J. Dis. Child.,* 141, 535, 1987.
34. Dietz, W. H., and Gordon, J. E., Obesity in infants, children and adolescents in the United States, *Nutr. Res.,* 1, 193, 1981.
35. Bull, N. L., Studies of dietary habits, food consumption and nutrient intakes of adolescents and young adults, *Wld. Rev. Nutr. Diet.,* 57, 24, 1988.
36. Amador, M., Ramos, L. T., Morono, M., and Hermelo, M. P., Growth rate reduction during energy restriction in obese adolescents, *Exp. Clin. Endocrinol.,* 96, 73, 1990.
37. Coates, T. J., and Hartung, C. E., Treating obesity in children and adolescents: a review, *Am. J. Public Health,* 68, 143, 1978.
38. Epstein, L. H., Valoski, A., Wing, R. R., and McCurley, J., Ten-year follow-up of behavioral, family based treatment for obese children, *JAMA,* 264, 251, 1990.
39. Sclafani, A., and Springer, D., Dietary obesity in adult rats: similarities to hypothalamic and human obesities, *Physiol. Behav.,* 17, 461, 1976.
40. Kendall A., Levitsky, D. A., Strupp, B. J., and Lissner, L., Weight loss on a low-fat diet: consequence of the imprecision of the control of food intake in humans, *Am. J. Clin. Nutr.,* 53, 1124, 1991.
41. Sheppard, L., Kristal, A. R., and Kushi, L. H., Weight loss in women participating in a randomized trial of low-fat diets, *Am. J. Clin. Nutr.,* 54, 821, 1991.
42. Drewnowski, A., The new fat replacements: a strategy for reducing fat consumption, *Postgrad. Med.,* 87, 1000, 1990.

# 12 Dietary Fat and the Control of Food Intake

**Barbara J. Rolls and David J. Shide**

Americans consume more fat than is currently recommended. Approximately 37% of their energy consumption is derived from fat despite frequent warnings that intakes of greater than 30% increase the risk of coronary disease, some types of cancer, and obesity.[1] In this chapter we examine research relevant to three hypotheses concerning why fat is overeaten: (1) fat increases the palatability of foods, (2) high-fat foods are energy dense and are overeaten because the volume of food eaten is maintained at a relatively constant level, and (3) high-fat foods are not as satiating as foods high in carbohydrate or protein.

## I. PALATABILITY OF FAT

Surveys of attitudes toward dietary fat indicate that intake of fat is related more to its perceived pleasantness than to its impact on health;[2,3] highly preferred foods often have a high fat content. Preference for fatty foods appears linked to fat's influences on the sensory qualities of foods. Odors and flavors of foods can depend on fat-soluble volatile flavor molecules;[4] fat also gives foods a variety of characteristic textures that make them highly palatable.[5] Since taste is the primary reason given for food selection,[6] fat preference will have a marked impact on nutrient and energy intakes. Low-fat diets are often found to be bland and monotonous so that individuals, even cardiac patients who should be highly motivated, find it difficult to maintain long-term compliance to them.[7]

Although it is presumed that sensory qualities of fat in foods promote overconsumption, there is little direct evidence for this. Several investigators have found that body weight is related to preferences for fat. Drewnowski and colleagues found that obese and formerly obese individuals preferred higher levels of fat in mixtures of dairy products and sugar than did lean individuals.[8] Mela and Sacchetti also found a positive relationship between sensory preferences for fat in a variety of foods and percent body fat in

0-8493-4466-2/94/$0.00+$.50

normal weight subjects.[9] However, it should be noted that within individuals the preferred level of fat varied widely between different types of foods. Also, the overall preferred level of fat in the diet did not correlate with the percent of fat being consumed by the subjects as determined by diet records. This lack of correlation may be methodological in that relatively few foods were given sensory ratings compared to the wide variety of foods being consumed.[9]

A variety of recently introduced fat substitutes and fat mimetics,[10] which retain fatty flavors in food, have provided new tools for studying fat intake. Whether the use of these products will affect fat intake and preferences for fat has yet to be determined. A critical question is whether individuals will learn with repeat consumption that these foods do not satisfy hunger as effectively as the full-fat versions of the foods. This is important because it may mean that the palatability of reduced-fat foods will fall so that they are no longer selected; alternatively it could mean that more of these foods or other foods in a meal will be consumed in order to satisfy hunger.

Clearly, more research is needed to understand how the sensory qualities of fat, and individual differences in preferences for dietary fat, influence human food intake and selection. Despite the paucity of information, it seems clear that fat enhances the palatability of a wide range of foods. As the palatability of high-fat foods appears linked to their high energy density,[11] the energy composition of foods could also influence food intake and selection.

## II. ENERGY DENSITY AND INTAKE

It is likely that both the energy content of foods and the weight or volume consumed interact to influence the amount eaten. The energy equivalents of the macronutrients based on the methods of Atwater are 9 kcal/g for fat and 4 kcal/g for carbohydrate and protein. Thus, if there is a tendency to maintain the volume or weight of food consumed at a constant level, high-fat diets will be associated with high energy intakes. Several studies indicate that the high energy density of fat is a factor in its overconsumption.

Most of the data relevant to the issue of energy density as a determinant of intake of high-fat foods come from measurements of amounts consumed when subjects were offered free access to high- or low-fat foods. One of the easiest ways to manipulate the fat content of the diet is to offer subjects fiber-rich starchy foods. With this kind of manipulation, a much larger volume of the low-fat foods must be consumed to achieve a given energy intake. Duncan and colleagues fed subjects a high-fiber, low-fat diet for 5 days and a high-fat diet of twice the energy density (0.7 vs. 1.5 kcal/g) for 5 days.[12] Individuals consumed the experimental diets in three meals and were allowed no other foods. Nearly twice as many calories were consumed during the high-energy density diet compared to the low-energy density diet (3000 vs. 1570 kcal daily). When subjects ate the low-energy density diet, they were slightly hungrier at meal times, but they found the meals satiating. Although the authors concluded that the energy content of the diet is not the sole or even the major determinant of satiety (at least in the short-term), they did not consider the possibility that the amount (weight or volume) consumed could have been a factor. By calculation, the subjects ate approximately 2243 g/day on the low-fat diet and 2000 g/day on the high-fat diet. Thus, although there was some increase in amount eaten in the low-energy density condition, the amount eaten daily was more constant than the energy consumed.[12]

Two other studies conducted at Cornell appear to confirm the relative constancy of the amount consumed when the fat content of the diet is altered. In the first of these studies,[13] females of varying body weight participated in a sequence of three 2-week dietary treatments in which 15 to 20, 30 to 35, or 45 to 50% of the energy was consumed as fat. Relative to their energy consumption on the medium-fat diet, which was considered the baseline, subjects spontaneously consumed an 11.3% energy deficit on the low-fat diet and a 15.4% surfeit on the high-fat diet, resulting in significant changes in body weight. There was a tendency to show some compensation for the energy deficit, reflected in differences in the weight of food consumed. Weighed-food intakes of subjects increased by 31 g/day (2.1%) on the low-fat diet and decreased by 53 g/day (3.7%) on the high-fat diet; overall, the amount of food consumed did not significantly differ between the high- (1412 g/day) and low-fat (1496 g/day) diets. Thus, across conditions the amount consumed apparently remained more constant than the energy intakes.[13] The relative constancy of the amount consumed was seen more clearly in the second study in which female subjects were allowed a low-fat diet (20–25% fat) or a control diet (35–40% fat) for 11 weeks each.[14] Although energy intake in the low-fat condition gradually increased over the 11 weeks, subjects showed a total caloric compensation of only 35% over the 11 weeks of the study. There were no significant differences in the grams of food consumed over the time of the study between the two conditions.

Another recent investigation suggests that the volume of food consumed is maintained when dietary fat is manipulated.[15] Subjects participated in two 2-day sessions, in which they consumed all their meals in the laboratory; they received low-fat foods during one session, high-fat (containing less than 25% energy from carbohydrate) during the other. As expected, energy intake was significantly higher when subjects consumed the high-fat foods. However, the total weight of food consumed in the two conditions did not differ significantly. This led the authors to suggest that daily energy intake was probably determined by fullness of the gastrointestinal tract and the energy density of the food.[15] Results from this study also supported the idea that subjects ate to maintain a critical level of carbohydrate in their diet, related to the rate of carbohydrate utilization. This raises the possibility that when carbohydrate levels are low in a high-fat diet, subjects may overeat in the attempt to derive necessary levels of carbohydrate.[15]

In all of these studies in which dietary fat was manipulated, subjects were given access only to foods of a particular energy density. In such situations there appears to be a tendency to eat a relatively constant amount of food. The control of food intake can be affected by preabsorptive factors such as the amount of chewing and swallowing required, as well as cognitive factors, i.e., the perceived fat content of a food, previous experiences with the satiety value of foods, or assessment of the amount of food on the plate. In support of cognitive influences, a recent study indicates that information about the fat content of a preload interacts with the actual caloric content to influence subsequent eating behavior.[16] Specifically, normal-weight females who received a yogurt labeled "low-fat" consumed more calories during a subsequent lunch meal than after an equicaloric yogurt labeled "high-fat".

The relative influence of the many factors affecting food intake will depend on the experimental paradigm. While in the experiments just described the amount of food consumed appears to be controlled more precisely than energy intake, in other experimental situations some humans demonstrate an ability to maintain a constant daily energy intake, even when the composition of the diet is varied markedly.

## III. PHYSIOLOGICAL CONTROL OF FAT INTAKE

Another hypothesis accounting for the overconsumption of dietary fat is that it is not as satiating as other nutrients;[17,18] this would relate to postabsorptive factors such as nutrient absorption, hormonal release, substrate utilization, and oxidation of nutrients. Evidence from several sources suggests that fat and carbohydrate have very different postingestional consequences. Data from experiments measuring postabsorptive metabolism suggest that dietary fat is not metabolized as rapidly after meals as carbohydrate and protein.[19] Ingested carbohydrates produce rapid rises in blood glucose[20] while fats often depress blood glucose.[21] Thus, it is possible that carbohydrates produce more rapid satiety than fats. On the other hand, some forms of dietary fat stimulate the release of cholecystokinin upon entering the intestine[22] and this putative satiety hormone[23] could, in theory, lead to early satiety. On the basis of these different physiological effects it can be argued that dietary fat is either more or less satiating than other macronutrients. A number of studies have been conducted to address potential differences in the satiating efficiencies of fat and carbohydrate.

## A. Intravenous Nutrients

One of the most controlled ways to investigate the effects of macronutrients is to infuse them directly into the stomach or vasculature. This bypasses the effects of taste or learned responses to foods. Such infusions (enteral or parenteral feeding) are common in hospital settings where oral intake is difficult. In a recent study, healthy males consumed only a liquid diet (Ensure®, Ross Laboratories, Columbus, OH) while confined to a metabolic ward for 16 to 19 days. When they were surreptitiously infused with a mixture of fat, glucose, and amino acids, they reduced intake by an amount that almost matched the infused calories. Subjects given only glucose reduced intake by 86% of the infused calories, whereas those given only fat showed a reduction in caloric intake equal to about 44% of infused calories. These results imply that the postabsorptive monitoring of carbohydrate is more accurate than that for fat and thus fats may be more satiating preabsorptively than postabsorptively.[17]

In a second study, responses to acute intravenous infusions of nutrients (500 kcal of either fat, carbohydrate, or normal saline), delivered over a 3.5-h period in the morning were determined; lean healthy males, who compensated for calories consumed orally, were examined. After intravenous infusions total caloric intake across the subsequent lunch and dinner meals (without calories provided by infusion) did not significantly differ between fat, carbohydrate, or saline conditions. No evidence for caloric compensation was found, suggesting that short-term intravenous nutrient infusions are less effective than oral preloads at suppressing subsequent caloric intake.[24] A study assessing responses to nutrients delivered intragastrically is currently in progress.

Although administering nutrients through intravenous and intragastric routes allows the study of mechanisms that may subserve food intake in humans, this situation is far removed from settings where normal eating behavior occurs. To study eating behavior in more naturalistic situations, a series of experiments have been conducted manipulating real foods in meal-to-meal and day-to-day settings.

## B. Preloads of Ordinary Fat: Five vs. Carbohydrate

Another way to test the hypothesis that fat has a different satiety value than other macronutrients is to give fixed preloads of nutrients or foods varying in nutrient composition and determine the effect on subsequent hunger, satiety, and food intake. The amount of fat can be varied either by replacing it with other nutrients or by incorporating a noncaloric fat substitute. Preloads must be matched for volume and for sensory characteristics, since as already discussed these factors could influence food intake. However, a number of studies have not controlled for both of these factors.[25-27]

Two recent studies meeting these criteria employed yogurt preloads varying in carbohydrate and fat levels, with similar sensory properties and energy densities, so that differences in the responses to the yogurts would depend on the physiological effects of the nutrients. In the first study, lean unrestrained males and females (for example, individuals who were not concerned with their body weight, as assessed by the cognitive restraint dimension of the Eating Inventory[28]) consumed preloads 30, 90, or 180 min before a self-selected lunch. There were no differences related to the level of carbohydrate or fat in the preloads on hunger, fullness, energy intake, or the types of foods or macronutrients consumed.[29] The fact that no differences were seen between fat or carbohydrate at either 30 or 180 min is important. At 30 min it is likely that the main influences on intake would be preabsorptive, whereas by 180 min postabsorptive factors would be expected to exert their control.[20]

A point that has not yet been emphasized is that individuals may vary markedly in their responses to fat manipulations. Individuals who are obese or who have a tendency to become obese may differ from lean individuals not only in their preference for high-fat foods, but also in their ability to adjust subsequent intake to compensate for consumption of high-fat, high-calorie foods. In the second preloading study[30] such potential individual differences were assessed by testing normal-weight and obese females who were either restrained (concerned or preoccupied with their body weight) or unrestrained, in addition to normal-weight restrained and unrestrained males. Subjects consumed yogurts with three different energy densities, which also varied in fat and carbohydrate composition, 30 min before a lunch meal in a repeated-measures dose-response design. There were some interesting differences between groups.

Normal-weight unrestrained males showed the best caloric compensation at lunch for the calories they received in the preload, with a mean of $99.1 \pm 2.3\%$ compensation averaged across the five preload conditions. This means that subjects accurately reduced subsequent intake at lunch meals in response to preloads of varying energy density. The fact that this group accurately compensated for yogurts varying in caloric density suggests that subjects are not responding solely on the basis of volume cues (yogurt volume was constant across conditions). In contrast, all three groups of restrained subjects showed little differential compensation for the preloads, such that they ate the same amounts following each preload.[30] Further studies are planned to determine whether restrained or obese individuals adopt the strategy of eating the same number of calories regardless of the

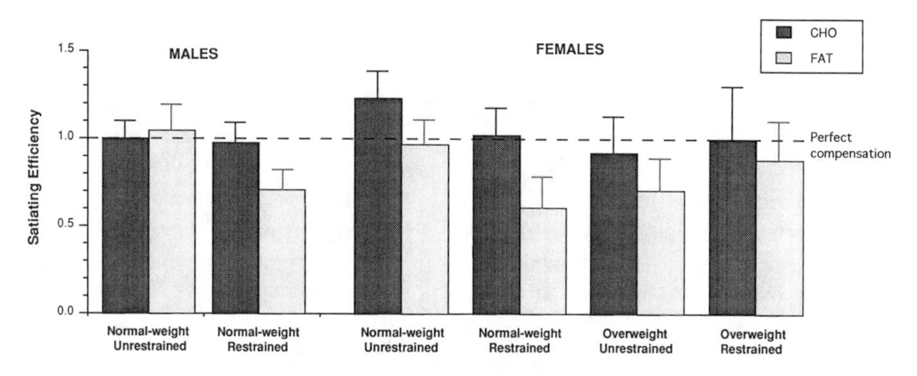


**FIGURE 1**. Satiating efficiencies for fat and carbohydrate (CHO) in the groups tested. Satiating efficiency is calculated as the negative slope of the regression line relating test meal intake to preload size. A satiating efficiency of 1 represents perfect compensation, i.e. test meal intake + preload intake = intake in the no load condition (KCAL).

energy content of a preload, which is related to an impaired ability to respond to physiological cues associated with food intake.

Across groups, fat in the yogurts was found to be less satiating than carbohydrate, i.e., subjects consumed more following preloads deriving most of their energy from fat relative to equicaloric preloads deriving most of their energy from carbohydrate. However, as show in Figure 1, the groups responded differently to the preloads; in normal weight unrestrained males, there was no tendency for fat to be less satiating than carbohydrate. By contrast, in all other groups the results reflected the overall finding. Thus, these preliminary findings suggest that some groups may be relatively insensitive to the satiety value of fat whereas others are not. Further investigation is required to specify the relationships between fat intake and individual differences.

Responses to macronutrient and energy manipulations have also been studied in longer-term experimental settings. In a residential study in which subjects were monitored continuously for 13 days, the carbohydrate or fat content of lunch on different days was varied by 400 kcal. Although commercially available foods were used, subjects were unable to detect the differences in the foods. Subjects were required to eat a standard lunch, but over the rest of the day could consume as much as they liked from a wide selection of foods that varied in energy and macronutrient density. When the caloric content of the lunch was reduced by 400 kcal of either carbohydrate or fat, subjects made up for the calories later in the day, so that daily energy intake remained constant across conditions.[31]

In a second residential study, the effects of greater covert manipulation of carbohydrate or fat content were assessed.[32] Daily energy intake during three required-eating occasions (breakfast, lunch, and afternoon snack) was varied by approximately 700 to 1700 kcal (22 to 53% of the baseline spontaneous intake when there was no required eating), and the effects on intake chosen from a wide variety of foods during the rest of the day were assessed. The results were similar to those of the previous residential study in that caloric compensation was seen, and there was no difference between carbohydrate and fat manipulations in the effects on subsequent intake. Also, despite the wide range of required intakes, total daily energy intake remained relatively constant — within 15% of baseline spontaneous intake.[32]

### C. Preloads Using the Fat Substitute Sucrose Polyester

Manipulation of daily fat intake in the studies discussed thus far was achieved using commercially available products, and involved substituting carbohydrate for fat. Another approach is to replace fat with a nonabsorbable fat substitute such as sucrose polyester. Sucrose polyester (SPE) has physical and organoleptic properties similar to fat, but since it is not digested or absorbed contributes no calories to the diet.[7] The use of SPE allows levels of fat-derived energy to be varied while preserving the bulk, appearance, texture, and sensory characteristics of food.

Recently, three short-term studies have examined the effects of SPE on eating behavior. Two of the studies, one in the in the United Kingdom[33] and one in the United States,[34] were conducted using a similar protocol in lean, nondieting young men. Sucrose polyester was covertly used to replace 0, 20, or 36 g of fat at breakfast, and food intake and ratings of hunger over the following 24 h were recorded. Data collected at both sites were similar and showed that consumption of SPE did not affect daily energy intake, although SPE was associated with a decrease in daily fat intake. There were no systematic differences in ratings of hunger and fullness between conditions. A similar study was conducted in 2- to 5-year-olds over a 2-day period.[35] Approximately 123 kcal of fat was replaced by SPE over the first part of the first day, and intake was recorded until the end of the second day. As in adults, ingestion of SPE rather than fat resulted in a significant reduction in overall fat intake, but was not associated with a decline in total energy intake.

In all the studies in which the fat content of the diet was altered covertly, normal-weight, unrestrained males showed an ability to adjust subsequent intake to compensate for the energy content of the preloads. Caloric compensation was accurate, regardless of whether the nutrient composition of foods was changed by substituting carbohydrate for fat or by replacing fat with SPE. However, the question of whether fat is overeaten because it is less satiating calorie-for-calorie than other macronutrients remains to be conclusively answered.

## IV. CONCLUSIONS

Normal-weight, nondieting individuals have the capacity to adjust energy intake appropriately in response to changes in the level of fat in foods. This ability is seen experimentally in preloading studies in which subjects are required to eat varying levels of fat and are then offered a wide variety of foods of different energy densities to consume. On the other hand, overconsumption of fat is seen in studies where individuals are offered only foods with a high-fat level. The addition of fat to foods makes them both more palatable and more energy dense. Thus, to show energy regulation subjects would have to eat a smaller amount of highly palatable foods, which they tend not to do. Subjects also typically fail to maintain the usual daily energy intake when they are offered only foods with a low-fat content. In this situation, they would have to eat greater amounts of foods that in general are not very palatable and that may be relatively unfamiliar; again they tend not to do this, although there is some indication that over time caloric compensation improves.[14]

It is clear from the studies reviewed here that energy intake in response to changes in the fat content of foods is modulated by a complex interplay of sensory factors, the amount or volume of food consumed, and physiological responses; the exact relation between these factors is affected by the experimental situation, and influenced by individual differences. To increase our understanding of ways to reduce fat intake, more studies systematically manipulating these three factors are needed to determine how energy and fat intakes are influenced in short- and long-term settings.

## ACKNOWLEDGMENTS

The authors of this article were supported by grants from the National Institutes of Health (DK-39177 and DK-40968).

## REFERENCES

1. National Research Council, *Diet and Health,* National Academy Press, Washington, D.C., 1989.
2. Shepherd, R., and Stockley, L., Fat consumption and attitudes towards food with a high-fat content, *Hum. Nutr.: Appl. Nutr.,* 39A, 431, 1985.
3. Shepherd, R., and Stockley, L., Nutrition knowledge, attitudes and fat consumption, *J. Am. Diet. Assoc.,* 87, 615, 1987.
4. Mela, D. J., The basis of dietary fat preferences, *Trends Food Sci. Technol.,* 1(3), 71, 1990.

5. Mela, D. J., Sensory preferences for fats: what, who, why?, *Food Qual. Pref.*, 2, 95, 1991.
6. Drewnowski, A., Fats and food acceptance: sensory, hedonic and attitudinal aspects. In: *Food Acceptance and Nutrition,* J. Solms, D. A. Booth, R. M. Pangborn, et al., Eds. Academic Press, New York, 1988, 189.
7. Drewnowski, A., The new fat replacements: a strategy for reducing fat consumption, *Postgrad. Med.,* 87, 111, 1990.
8. Drewnowski, A., Kurth, C. L., and Rahaim, J. E., Taste preferences in human obesity: environmental and familial factors, *Am. J. Clin. Nutr.,* 54, 635, 1991.
9. Mela, D. J., and Sacchetti, D. A., Sensory preferences for fats: relationships with diet and body composition, *Am. J. Clin. Nutr.,* 53, 908, 1991.
10. Schlicker, S. A., and Regan, C., Innovations in reduced-calorie foods: a review of fat and sugar replacement technologies, *Top. Clin. Nutr.,* 6, 50, 1990.
11. Johnson, S. L., McPhee, L., and Birch, L. L., Conditioned preferences: young children prefer flavors associated with high dietary fat, *Physiol. Behav.,* 50, 1245, 1991.
12. Duncan, K. H., Bacon, J. A., and Weinsier, R. L., The effects of high and low energy density diets on satiety, energy intake, and eating time of obese and nonobese subjects, *Am. J. Clin. Nutr.,* 37, 763, 1983.
13. Lissner, L., Levitsky, D. A., Strupp, B. J., Kalkwarf, H. J., and Roe, D. A., Dietary fat and the regulation of energy intake in human subjects, *Am. J. Clin. Nutr.,* 46, 886, 1987.
14. Kendall, A., Levitsky, D. A., Strupp, B. J., and Lissner, L., Weight loss on a low-fat diet: consequence of the imprecision of the control of food intake in humans, *Am. J. Clin. Nutr.,* 53, 1124, 1991.
15. Tremblay, A., Lavallee, N., Almeras, N., Allard, L., Despres, J., and Bouchard, C., Nutritional determinants of the increase in energy intake associated with a high-fat diet, *Am. J. Clin. Nutr.,* 53, 1134, 1991.
16. Rolls, B. J., Shide, D. J., Hoeymans, N., Jas, P., and Nichols, A., Information about fat content of preloads influences energy intake in women, *Appetite,* 19, 123, 1992 (abstract).
17. Friedman, M. I., Gil, K. M., Rothkopf, M. M., and Askanazi, J., Postabsorptive control of food intake in humans, *Appetite,* 7, 258, 1986.
18. Gil, K. M., Skeie, B., Kvetan, V., Askanazi, J., and Friedman, M. I., Parenteral nutrition and oral intake: effect of glucose and fat infusions, *J. Parenter. Enteral. Nutr.,* 4, 426, 1991.
19. Schutz, Y., Flatt, J. P., and Jequier, E., Failure of dietary fat intake to promote fat oxidation: a factor favoring the development of obesity, *Am. J. Clin. Nutr.,* 50, 307, 1989.
20. Van Amelsvoort, J. M. M., Van Stratum, P., Kraal, J. H., Lussenburg, R. N., and Houtsmuller, U. M. T., Effects of varying the carbohydrate:fat ratio in a hot lunch on postprandial variables in male volunteers, *Br. J. Nutr.,* 61, 267, 1989.

21. McHugh, P. R., Moran, T. H., and Barton, G. N., Satiety: a graded behavioral phenomenon regulating caloric intake, *Science,* 190, 167, 1975.
22. Cantor, P., Cholecystokinin in plasma, *Digestion,* 42, 181, 1989.
23. Smith, G. P., and Gibbs, J., The satiating effect of cholecystokinin. In: *Control of Appetite,* M. Winick, Ed. John Wiley, New York, 1988, 35.
24. Shide, D. J., Caballero, B., Friedman, M., Moran, T. H., and Rolls, B. J., Differential effects of intravenous or oral nutrients on caloric intake in healthy humans, *Am. J. Clin. Nutr.,* 55 (Suppl.), 119, 1992.
25. de Graaf, C., Hulshof, T., Westrate, J. A., and Jas, P., Short-term effects of different amounts of protein, fats, and carbohydrates on satiety, *Am. J. Clin. Nutr.,* 55, 33, 1992.
26. Hill, A. J., Leathwood, P. D, and Blundell, J. E., Some evidence for short-term caloric compensation in normal weight human subjects: the effects of high-and-low-energy meals on hunger, food preference and food intake, *Hum. Nutr.: Appl. Nutr.,* 41A, 244, 1987.
27. Rolls, B. J., Hetherington, M., and Burley, V. J., The specificity of satiety: the influence of foods of different macronutrient content on the development of satiety, *Physiol. Behav.,* 43(a), 145, 1988.
28. Stunkard, A. J., and Messick, S., The three-factor eating questionnaire to measure dietary restraint, disinhibition, and hunger, *J Psychosom. Res.,* 29, 71, 1985.
29. Rolls, B. J., Kim, S., McNelis, A. L., Fischman, M. W., Foltin, R. W., and Moran, T. H., Time course of effects of preloads high in fat or carbohydrate on food intake and hunger ratings in humans, *Am. J. Physiol.,* 260, R756, 1991.
30. Rolls, B. J., Kim, S., Fischman, M. W., et al., Food intake following preloads of fat and carbohydrate in normal weight and obese individuals, Obes. Res., 1, 11S, 1992. (abstract).
31. Foltin, R. W., Fischman, M. W., Moran, T. H., Rolls, B. J., and Kelly, T. H., Caloric compensation for lunches varying in fat and carbohydrate content by humans in a residential laboratory, *Am. J. Clin. Nutr.,* 52, 969, 1990.
32. Foltin, R. W., Rolls, B. J., Moran, T. H., Kelly, T. H., McNelis, A. L., and Fischman, M. W., Caloric, but not macronutrient, compensation by humans for required-eating occasions with meals and snack varying in fat and carbohydrate, *Am. J. Clin. Nutr.,* 55, 331, 1992.
33. Burley, V. J., and Blundell, J. E., Evaluation of the action of a non-absorbable fat on appetite and energy intake in lean, healthy males, Int. J. Obes., 15 (Suppl. 1), 8, 1991 (abstract).
34. Rolls, B. J., Pirraglia, P. A., Jones, M. B., and Peters, J. C., Effects of olestra, a non-caloric fat substitute, on daily energy and fat intake in lean men, *Am. J. Clin. Nutr.,* 56, 84, 1992.
35. Birch, L. L., Johnson, S. J., Jones, M. B., and Peters, J. C., Effects of olestra, a non-caloric fat substitute, on children's energy and macronutrient intake. *Am. J. Clin. Nutr.,* in press.

# 13 Imprecise Control of Food Intake on Low-Fat Diets

**David A. Levitsky and Barbara J. Strupp**

The precision with which humans adjust their caloric intake in response to changes in the fat composition of the diet has important ramifications for the theory and practice of weight control. If the control of caloric intake is accurately regulated, then any attempt to reduce body weight by consuming more low-fat foods and less high-fat foods or by using fat substitutes would be futile because reducing caloric consumption would only cause an increase in food consumption. On the other hand, if eating behavior is not highly regulated, then it should not only be possible to lose weight by reducing the fat consumption alone (without "dieting"), but the weight loss should be maintained for as long as a person continues to eat a low-fat diet.

Such an approach to weight control is a clear alternative to current methods of weight control, which require voluntary restriction of the amount of food consumed. Such alternatives to conventional weight loss methods are desperately needed because current treatments are ineffective at producing a sustained weight loss.[1-3]

## I. STUDYING EATING BEHAVIOR IN THE LABORATORY

To examine the degree of precision to which humans calorically compensate for changes in dietary fat, one must have a valid and sensitive system for measuring human food intake. But how does one study the precision of the control of food intake in humans? At first glance, it appears easy. One merely has to put a human in front of a meal and weigh the amount of food consumed. However, it is possible that eating behavior studied in the laboratory may bear little resemblance to the kind of behavior that occurs outside the laboratory. Certainly, eating in a strange laboratory dining room surrounded by people in white coats is quite different from eating comfortably at home.

Because of the importance of validating the laboratory method of observing human feeding behavior, our first human study addressed this

0-8493-4466-2/94/$0.00+$.50

issue by assessing how well eating in the laboratory approximates eating outside the laboratory.[4] For this study, we trained a group of male and female volunteers ranging in age from 21 to 39 years to record their own weighed intakes. The study consisted of two 1-week blocks in which the subjects measured and recorded everything they ate from Monday through Thursday. During the first week the subjects ate in their homes. In the second week, subjects consumed only food prepared and served in the Cornell Clinical Nutrition Unit. Morning body weights were taken at the beginning and end of each 4-day block. Subjects were instructed to maintain the same activity pattern during week 2 as week 1.

The procedure we followed in the laboratory for feeding subjects for all of our studies of human feeding behavior requires the subjects to serve themselves from a buffet table. Most of the foods are offered as mixtures, e.g., casseroles, stir-fries, soups, and salads. When individual items are offered they are prepared in very small units requiring the subjects to take more than one unit to constitute a serving. Such a procedure was followed because humans tend to eat the amount of food that is placed on their plate[5] and we desired to provide subjects with as much opportunity as possible to determine their own intake.

Figure 1 shows the regression between mean caloric intake consumed over the 4-day block for each subject eating in the laboratory and eating at home. Three points are apparent. First, the amount of calories consumed in the laboratory is roughly equivalent to that consumed under more natural conditions. The correlation coefficient is 0.79 ($p < 0.01$). Second, although mean intake of the two conditions was not statistically different, the intercept of the regression indicates that subjects ate approximately 590 fewer calories in the laboratory than they ate outside the laboratory. People tend to eat slightly less in a laboratory setting than at home. Finally, the slope of the function was 0.80, indicating that the larger the eater (and probably, the bigger the person[6]), the greater the decrement in caloric intake when intake is measured in the laboratory.

Thus, although people eat slightly less food in the laboratory than they do under free conditions, the stability of the rank order of caloric intakes suggests that meaningful measures of human food intake can be obtained within the confines of a laboratory. We have used the laboratory method of studying human food intake under a variety of conditions[4] and found the measures to be both highly reliable and sensitive to many variables that affect feeding behavior when the unit of measurement of intake is total intake accumulated in blocks of 4 to 7 days. Using 7-day caloric intakes as the unit of analysis has enabled us to detect significant effects of such subtle variables as food fiber[7] and menstrual cycling.[8] With blocks of intake less than 4 days the variability of daily caloric intake is too great to detect these kinds of effects.

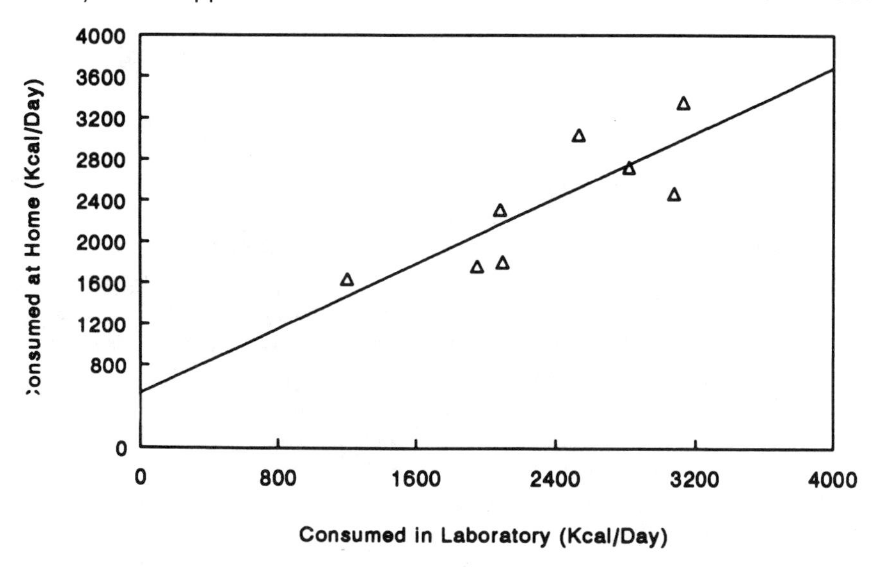


**FIGURE 1.** Correlation between daily caloric intake consumed in the laboratory and that eaten at home.

## II. EFFECT OF DIETARY FAT ON CALORIC INTAKE: A SHORT-TERM STUDY

Our first study of the role of dietary fat on caloric intake in humans[8] examined three levels of dietary fat. Each treatment lasted for 2 weeks and was presented in a balanced order. Each subject was tested under all three fat conditions. Within each condition the fat content of all foods contained about the same amount of fat. Thus for the high-fat conditions, the percent of calories from fat ranged from 45 to 50%, for the medium fat conditions all foods contained between 30 and 35% calories from fat, and for the low-fat conditions, the food consisted of 15 to 20% fat. Our rationale for making all the foods within a condition contain about the same percentage of calories as fat was that we did not want the subjects to change the amount of fat consumed by changing the foods they elected to eat under the various conditions. Using the uniform food method, no matter what foods the subjects chose they would remain within their designated fat content.

The foods used in the study were common foods such as muffins, cheese and tomato sandwiches, fruit yogurts, Waldorf salads, and macaroni, and offered on a 7-day rotation diet. All three versions of the foods (high-, medium-, and low-fat) were pretested and found to be equally as acceptable. The subjects sampled the foods before the study and were selected for the study only if they had no aversions to the foods.

Potential subjects completed a medical history, an eating restraint scale, and a 4-day food record. Only those females having no current medical problems, low restraint scores, regular eating patterns, at least 101% of the 1959 Metropolitan Life Insurance standards, and whose motivation for volunteering appeared to be more of wanting to be involved in nutritional research rather than for the money were accepted as subjects. The subjects were paid $7.50 per day and were given a bonus of an additional $7.50 per day if they completed the study. Subjects were told that the purpose of the study was to learn about the control of food intake in humans and were instructed to eat as much or as little as they desired. They were told to "listen to their bodies" to determine how much and what food to select and eat.

The study utilized a Latin square design and was run in two replications. Each subject received each level of fat for a 2-week period with order being counterbalanced. The data were analyzed using blocks of weekly intakes, although for presentation the data are represented as daily intakes per person. The analysis of intake data in blocks of 1 week produces sufficient statistical power to detect a 7% difference in caloric intake with a sample size of 24. The results of the study were quite clear as indicated in Figure 2. Daily intake was directly related to the percent of total calories consumed as fat: the higher the fat content of the foods, the greater the total calories consumed.

Figure 3 displays the mean daily intake across the 14 days of each dietary treatment. Each function was statistically flat (slope - 0, $p > 0.05$) indicating that the amount of calories the subjects consumed on the first day of each dietary treatment was maintained throughout the testing period. Thus, we found no evidence that humans adjust their daily caloric intake in response to changes in the fat content of the diet. Consequently, subjects exhibited a significant increase in mean body weight when consuming the high-fat diet ($p < 0.05$) and a loss in body weight when they consumed the low-fat diet ($p < 0.05$).

It is possible that despite our attempt at equating the various diets for acceptability at the beginning of the study, the subjects preferred the high-fat foods. However, the actual amount of food consumed of the high-fat diet was not significantly different (1412 vs. 1496 g/day) from the low-fat diet. Moreover, food palatability ratings taken during the course of the study revealed no statically significant difference in acceptability of the diets (2.63 for low-fat vs. 2.48 for the high-fat diet rated on a five-point scale). Thus, the increase in caloric consumption of the high-fat diet can be attributed only to an insensitivity of those mechanisms involved in the control of feeding behavior in humans when confronted with changes in dietary fat.

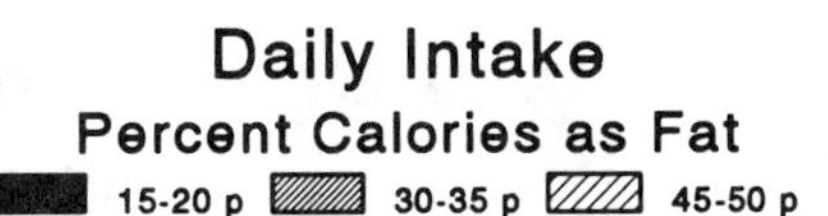


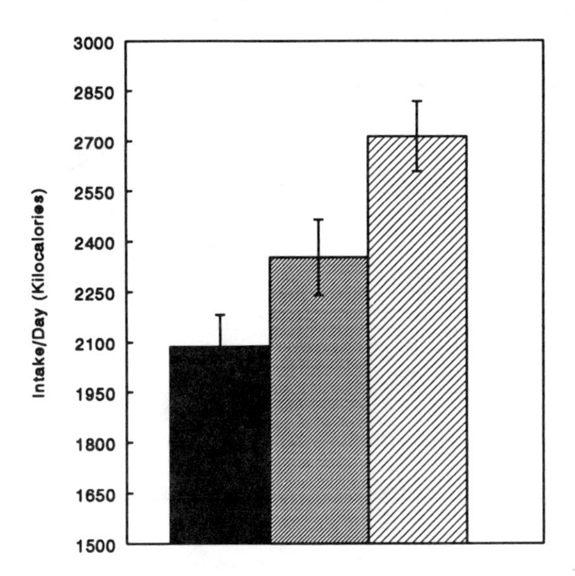


**FIGURE 2.** Mean and SE of caloric intake of subjects consuming foods consisting of low (15–20), medium (30–35), or high (45–50) percent of total calories as fat.

## III. EFFECT OF DIETARY FAT ON CALORIC INTAKE: A LONG-TERM STUDY

Although the results of the previous study showed quite clearly that humans do not show any caloric adjustment to changes in the fat content of the diet, it might be argued that 2 weeks is not sufficient time to allow the physiological controls of food intake to be expressed. Moreover, if we intend to use this information to suggest a therapy for reducing body weight, we require longer term studies of caloric compensation than a 2-week testing period. The next study attempted to fill this void by examining the effects of dietary fat on caloric intake measured over an 11-week interval.[9]

The basic procedure used was very similar to the previous study except that only two dietary conditions were used: a diet containing between 20 and 25% of total calories as fat, and a diet containing 35 to 40% fat. We chose the lower value on the basis that 25% fat is about as low a fat level Americans can consume without drastically limiting the kinds of foods they usually eat. The other change from the previous study is that the length of

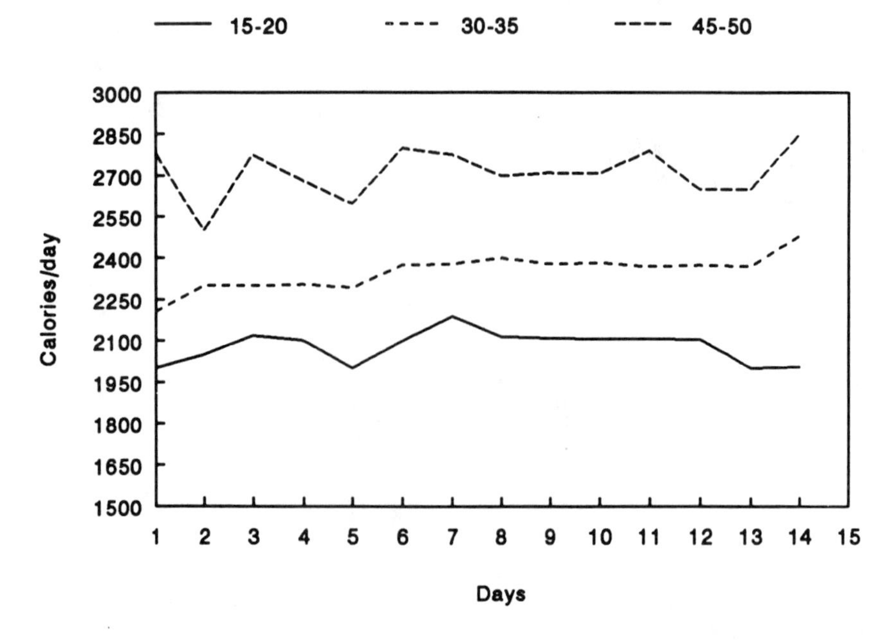


**FIGURE 3.** Mean daily caloric intake of subjects consuming foods consisting of low (15–20), medium (30–35), or high (45–50) percent of total calories as fat across 14 days of treatment.

time the subjects remained on each diet was 11 weeks rather than 2. A cross-over design was used with a 4-week "wash-out" time imposed between treatments. Thirteen of the 16 original subjects completed the study.

The results of this study are depicted in Figure 4. There was a slow but constant increase in caloric intake during the course of the 11-week observation period. The increase in slope of caloric intake function for the low-fat condition was statistically different from 0, but the change in the control condition was not. Consequently, it appears that some caloric compensation for the low-fat diet was occurring over the 11-week interval, though the compensation was weak and incomplete. By the end of 11 weeks the daily caloric intake from the low-fat diet was approximately 200 calories less than on the control diet. Overall difference in caloric intake between the two dietary treatments was statistically significant. Extrapolation from the two functions presented in Figure 4 suggests that complete caloric compensation might have occurred by 22 weeks.

Despite the fact that the difference in caloric intake between the low-fat and control diet conditions appeared to be decreasing, there was no indication

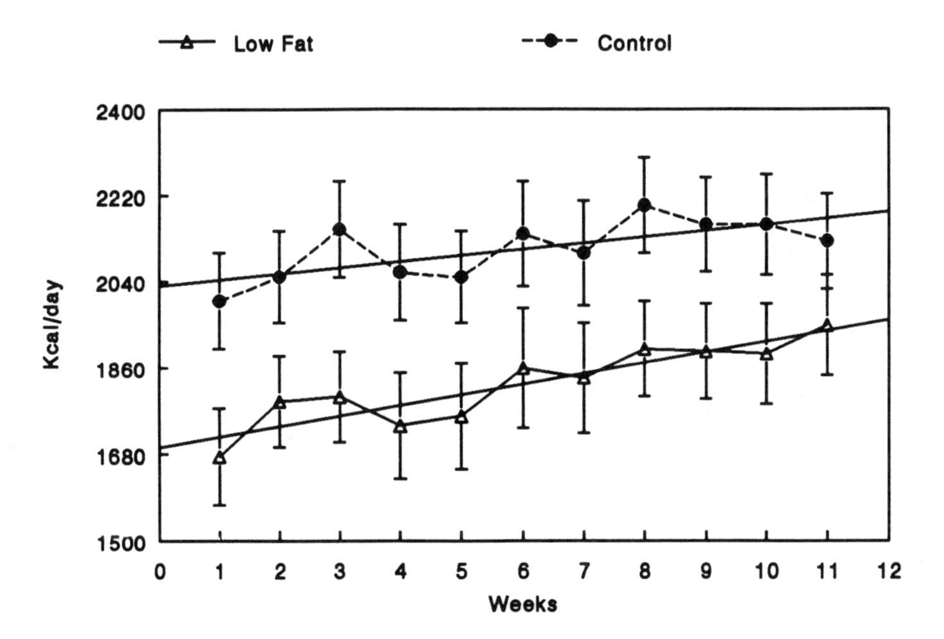


**FIGURE 4.** Mean and SE of daily caloric intake of subjects consuming foods consisting of low (20–25) or control (30–35) percent of total calories as fat averaged over the 11 weeks of treatment.

that the difference in body weight would collapse. Figure 5 shows the loss of body weight across the 11 weeks of each dietary condition. Subjects in both conditions lost weight throughout each dietary condition, supporting our original finding that people eat less in the laboratory than they would under more natural conditions. However, the subjects lost significantly more weight when consuming the low-fat diet than the control diet. Moreover, there is no indication that body weight on the low-fat diet would increase to the level they reached on the control diet.

## IV. EFFECT OF DIETARY FAT ON CALORIC INTAKE: A COMMUNITY STUDY

One might argue, however, that it is easy for people to lose weight on a low-fat diet when other people are preparing the food and that people might not lose weight under more natural conditions where they had to prepare their own food and in an environment in which their natural preference for high-fat foods would

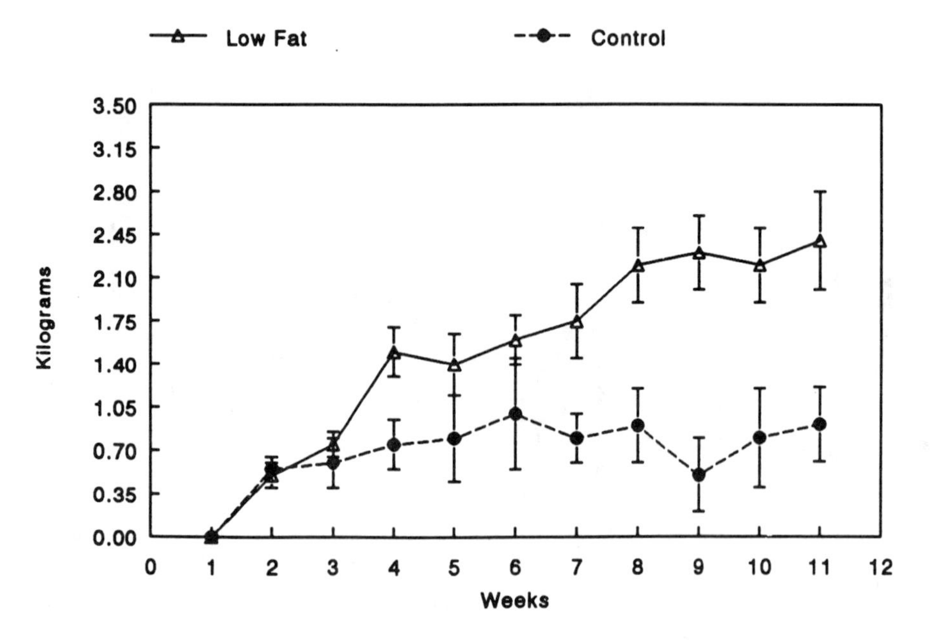


**FIGURE 5.** Mean and SE of loss in body weight of subjects consuming foods consisting of low (20–25) or control (30–35) percent of total calories as fat averaged over the 11 weeks of treatment.

cause them to easily deviate from their diet. To examine these hypotheses, we designed a community study in which we recruited 48 women from the Ithaca community. We screened the subjects using the same criteria we used for the previous study.[9] We told the subjects that the purpose of the study was to examine the relationship between what people were eating and blood lipids and taught everyone how to record 4-day (Wednesday to Saturday) weighed food intakes.

After analyzing the first 4-day food record, we divided the subjects into two groups matched on the basis of their daily fat intake. We informed one group (the low-fat group) of all the health hazards of ingesting a high-fat diet. All subjects continued taking 4-day weighed food records for the next 3 weeks. The reason the control group was also instructed to take weighed food intakes was that food weighing and recordkeeping affects what one eats and because we wanted to learn whether eating a low-fat diet can cause weight loss, we had to eliminate the effect of recordkeeping as a possible confounding variable. We neither defined the level of dietary fat that constituted a low-fat diet nor told the subjects how to estimate the fat content of foods.

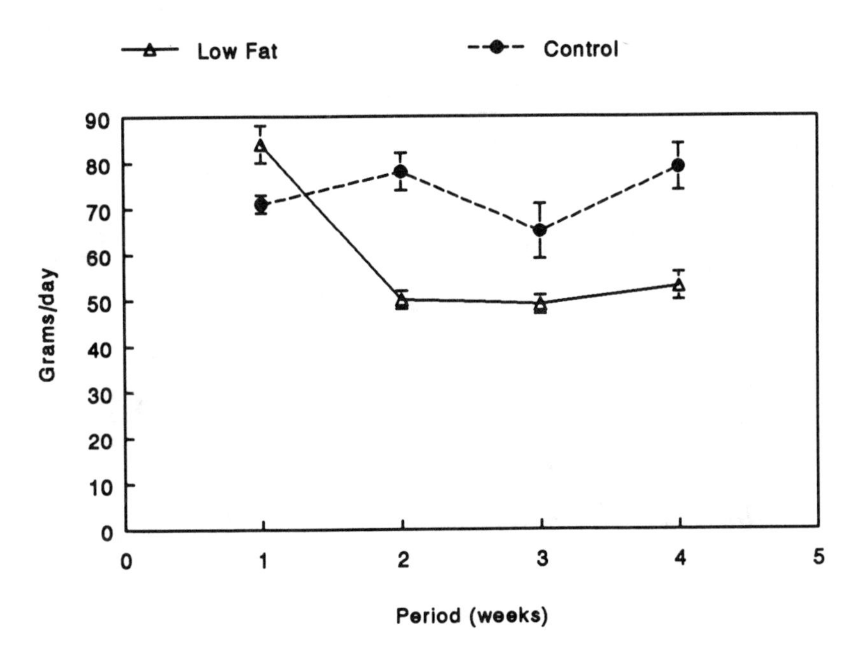


**FIGURE 6.** Mean and SE of daily fat intake of subjects instructed to consume a low-fat diet and controls averaged over the 4 weeks of the study.

Figure 6 shows the mean daily intake of fat calculated over the 4 weeks of the study. Clearly, when instructed to restrict dietary fat, subjects preparing their own meals can comply, at least within a 3-week period. What is most interesting is that expressed as a percentage, subjects reduced their intake to about 25% of total calories. Because the intake of neither carbohydrate nor protein changed significantly, total caloric intake was significantly ($p < 0.05$) reduced for the experimental group by about 250 kcal/day. As can be seen in Figure 7, the consequence of these changes resulted in significantly more weight lost by the experimental group than the controls. From the analysis of the diaries, no changes in life style other than the change in diet could account for this loss in body weight.

## V. SIGNIFICANCE OF FINDING FOR PROBLEM OF WEIGHT CONTROL

The results of all three studies clearly indicate that humans exhibit very poor caloric compensation for the changes in dietary fat within the range of from 20 to about 40% of total calories. These results are consistent with

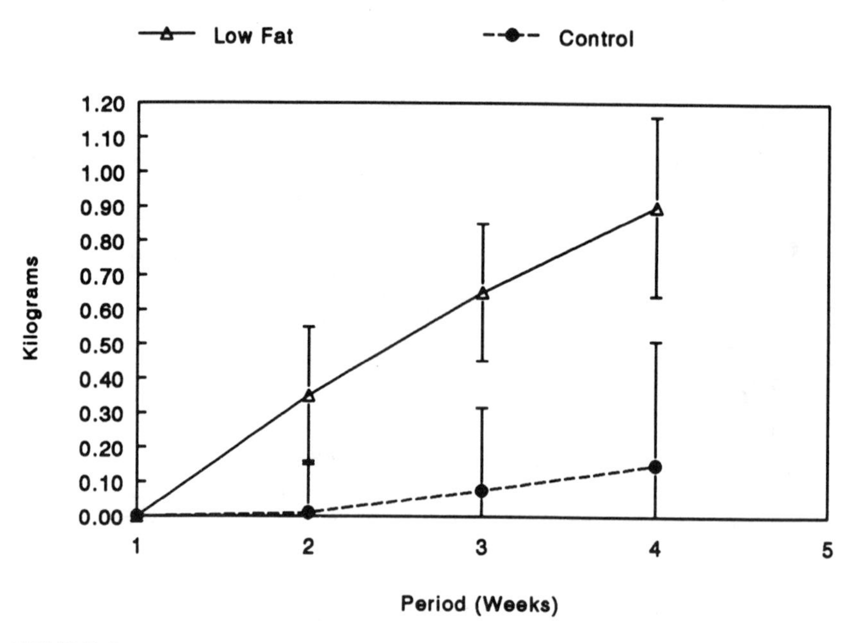


**FIGURE 7.** Mean and SE of loss in body weight of subjects instructed to consume a low-fat diet and controls averaged over the 4 weeks of the study.

other studies of human food intake,[10,11] although they appear to be at variance with the studies of Foltin and Rolls and their associates.[12,13] Foltin et al.[12,13] observed almost complete (80–85%) caloric compensation occurred within a 24-h period following the ingestion of either a high-carbohydrate or high-fat lunch. There are two possible explanations for this apparent discrepancy between the Foltin and Rolls group and our results. First, the Foltin group confined their subjects to an isolated environment for the duration of the study — lasting usually 6 or 7 days. Because such an isolated environment eliminates the myriad of factors that may influence feeding behavior in more natural environments, their subjects may have had a greater opportunity to be influenced by physiological cues associated with energy balance than ours. The subjects in our studies were not confined, but maintained their normal working activities, except for eating. Such differences raise serious questions, however, as to the practical importance of these putative physiological cues for the maintenance of body weight if they can be so easily overridden by normal activities.

A second reason for the disparity in findings between the Foltin and Rolls group and ours may lie in the selection of subjects. The Foltin and Rolls group[12,13] typically used lean young males, while we utilized slightly overweight females. There is evidence that lean young men display better caloric compensation than do females. Porikos and her co-workers[14,15] found normal-weight young men displayed statistically significant, yet only modest caloric compensation (40%) in response to a reduction in dietary carbohydrate, whereas obese women showed virtually no compensation for the identical dietary manipulation.

It is interesting to note, however, that in a recent paper by the Foltin and Rolls group[16] in which they utilized basically the same kind of testing situation as their previous studies, they observed no caloric compensation in humans consuming a diet composed of 17% of calories as fat and one consisting of 44% calories as fat. They described these diets as low- and medium-fat diets, respectively, and these correspond to our low- and high-fat diets. Caloric compensation was observed, however, when their subjects consumed a very high-fat diet composed of 58% of calories as fat.

Thus, taken together, the data on the human response to altered dietary fat suggest that effective alternatives to the traditional "low-calorie diet" as a means of producing a sustained reduction in body weight are possible. Our data show quite clearly that the ability of humans to adjust their eating behavior to compensate for changes in dietary fat between the ranges of 20 to 40% of calories appears to be quite poor. Even when some caloric compensation occurs, there is no indication that body weight (fat) will return to predietary change levels. The consequence of this research is that it should be possible to produce sustained loss in body weight without the need to count calories or limit portion sizes, but merely by reducing dietary fat alone.

## REFERENCES

1. Wing, R. R., and Jeffrey, R. W., Outpatient treatments of obesity: a comparison of methodology and clinical results, *Int. J. Obes.,* 3, 261, 1979.
2. Stunkard, A. J., Behavioral treatment of obesity: the current status, *Int. J. Obes.,* 2, 237, 1978.
3. Bennett, W., Dietary treatments of obesity, *Ann. N.Y. Acad. Sci.,* 499, 250, 1987.
4. Obarzanek, E., and Levitsky, D. A., Eating in the laboratory: is it representative?, *Am. J. Clin. Nutr.,* 42, 323, 1985.
5. Siegel, P. S., The completion compulsion in human eating, *Psychol. Rep.,* 3, 15, 1957.
6. Lissner, L., Stevens, J., Levitsky, D. A., Rasmussen, K. M., and Strupp, B. J., Variations in energy intake during the menstrual cycle: implications for food-intake research, *Am. J. Clin. Nutr.,* 48, 956, 1988.

7. Stevens, J. A., Levitsky, D. A., Van Soest, P. J., Roberson, J. B., Kalkwarf, H. J., and Roe, D. A., Effect of psyllium gum and wheat bran on spontaneous energy intake, *Am. J. Clin. Nutr.,* 16, 812, 1987.
8. Lissner, L., Levitsky, D. A., Strupp, B. J., et al., Dietary fat and the regulation of energy intake in human subjects, *Am. J. Clin. Nutr.,* 46, 886, 1987.
9. Kendall-Casella, A., Levitsky, D. A., Strupp, B. J., and Lissner, L., Weight loss on a low-fat diet: consequence of the imprecision of the control of food intake in humans, *Am. J. Clin. Nutr.,* 53, 1124, 1991.
10. Glueck, C. J., Hastings, M. M., Allen, C., et al., Sucrose polyester and covert caloric dilution, *Am. J. Clin. Nutr.,* 35, 1352, 1982.
11. Duncan, K. H., Bacon, J. A., and Weinsier, R. L., The effects of high and low energy density diets on satiety, energy intake, and eating time of obese and nonobese subjects, *Am. J. Clin. Nutr.,* 37, 763, 1983.
12. Foltin, R. W., Fischman, M. W., Emurian, C. S., and Rachlinski, J. J., Compensation for calorie dilution in humans given unrestricted access to food in a residential laboratory, *Appetite,* 10, 13, 1988.
13. Foltin, R. W., Fischman, M. W., Moran, T. H., Rolls, B. J., and Kelly, T. H., Caloric compensation for lunches varying in fat and carbohydrate content by humans in a residential laboratory, *Am. J. Clin. Nutr.,* 52, 969, 1990.
14. Porikos, K. P., Booth, G., and Van Ittalie, T. B., Effects of covert nutritive dilution on the spontaneous food intake of obese individuals: a pilot study, *Am. J. Clin. Nutr.,* 30, 1968, 1977.
15. Porikos, K. P., Hesser, M. F., and Van Ittalie, T. B., Caloric regulation in normal weight men maintained on a palatable diet of conventional foods, *Physiol. Behav.,* 29, 293, 1982.
16. Foltin, R. W., Rolls, B. J., Moran, T. H., Kelly, T. H., McNelis, A. L., and Fishchman, M. W., Caloric, but not macronutrient, compensation by humans for required-eating occasions with meals and snack varying in fat and carbohydrate, *Am. J. Clin. Nutr.,* 55, 331, 1992.

# 14 Dietary Fiber: Does It Affect Food Intake and Body Weight?

**Allen S. Levine and Charles J. Billington**

## I. INTRODUCTION

A low-fiber diet may be associated with a variety of diseases of Western Societies, including cancer, heart disease, diabetes, and several diseases of the gastrointestinal tract.[1] Those societies in which a diet naturally high in fiber is consumed do not have an obese population. This has led to the suggestion that dietary fiber may be useful in the treatment of obesity. In the present review, we will summarize those studies that have addressed the utility of dietary fiber in the treatment of obesity.

In 1974 Trowell defined dietary fiber as "remnants of plant cells resistant to hydrolysis by the alimentary enzymes of man, the group of substances that remain in the ileum but are partly hydrolyzed by bacteria in the colon."[2] Dietary fibers have been classified by water solubility; soluble fibers being those that form gels including gums, pectins, and mucilages.[1] Cellulose, lignin, and certain hemicelluloses are classified as insoluble fibers. Naturally occurring fibers present in foods generally contain a mixture of both types of fiber, some being more concentrated in soluble or insoluble. For example, apples are concentrated in soluble fiber and wheat bran contains more insoluble fiber.

There are many reasons to believe that fiber could reduce food intake and help control body weight (Table 1). High-fiber foods take longer to eat.[3] For example, a low-fiber food such as apple juice can be ingested more rapidly than a relatively high-fiber apple. Guar gum and pectin slow gastric emptying, which may promote a sense of fullness for a longer period of time.[4] Fiber is thought to reduce the digestibility of food by approximately 2 to 4%.[5,6] This results in increased fecal loss of energy, which could alter effective energy intake. Soluble dietary fiber has been reported to alter some

0-8493-4466-2/94/$0.00+$.50

**TABLE 1**
**Why Dietary Fiber Might Alter Food Intake and Body Weight**

| |
|---|
| Takes longer to ingest high-fiber foods |
| Some fiber types decrease the rates of gastric emptying and transit time through the small intestine |
| Decrease in the digestibility and absorption of foods |
| Release of GI hormones that affect food intake |

GI hormones. Since many GI hormones are known to alter food intake, it is possible that fiber-induced release of peptides might lead to a change in feeding behavior.

Based on the above observations, it seems likely that dietary fiber might influence food intake and hence body weight. Many studies, using a variety of fiber types, have been conducted.[7-10] These include studies with high-fiber foods, with fiber isolates, or with fiber isolates added to food. Open trial, blind, and double blind studies have been reported using both parallel and crossover designs for various time periods ranging from one meal to months. Food intake, hunger, and/or body weight have been the dependent measures in these studies. In some studies subjects were either obese or undergoing weight loss regimens, whereas in others subjects were normal-weight volunteers. Thus, it is difficult to simply answer the question: does dietary fiber result in a decrease in body weight and food intake?

One of the earliest trials evaluating the effect of fiber on food intake was conducted by Yudkin in 1959.[11] A group of obese women was given a preload of methylcellulose before each meal. The women ingesting 10 g/day of methylcellulose lost 4.5 kg over the 6-week period, whereas the control group lost 2.8 kg. Unfortunately, this trial was not blinded or placebo controlled. Also, food intake was not monitored in this study. Since this study, 50 studies have been reported concerning the effects of dietary fiber on food intake and body weight. These data have been summarized in four excellent reviews, two by Blundell and Burley,[8,9] one by Stevens,[7] and a report prepared for the Food and Drug Administration.[10]

## II. SHORT-TERM FIBER TRIALS

We will first address those studies in which fiber was given once or twice, either as a preload or part of meal. Thirteen studies of this type were conducted.[3,12-23] Ten of these studies found that fiber either reduced food intake or decreased hunger. Most of these studies were conducted in normal-weight volunteers. Porikos and Hagamen[22] studied the effects of a preload of methylcellulose on food intake in normal and obese subjects. The high fiber (6.6 g dietary fiber) preload decreased food intake in the 19 obese subjects, but not in the 50 normal subjects. The three negative studies were also conducted in normal subjects.[12,14,16] A variety of sources of fiber or foods high in fiber decreased food intake or hunger, including guar gum, wheat bran, methylcellulose, breakfast cereals, fruits, and high-fiber pasta. The effective doses of dietary fiber ranged from as low as 2 g (guar gum)[23] to as high as 22 g (wheat fiber).[21] Some studies used foods naturally high in fiber, whereas others used foods supplemented with fiber. None of the acute studies used tablets containing isolated fiber alone. Haber et al.[3] evaluated the effect of whole apples, pureed apples, or apple juice on satiety when consumed in isocaloric amounts. The juice was the least satiating and the whole fruit the most satiating. Bolton et al.[13] found the same effect with whole grapes or oranges compared to the juices of these fruits. Burley et al.[15] fed subjects higher fiber foods (30 g) at lunch and found that food intake was decreased following lunch until bedtime. Levine et al.[21] found that ingestion of breakfast cereals that contained concentrated amounts of wheat bran decreased food intake during lunch. When subjects ingested a low-fiber cereal (Post Toasties)™ they ate 891 kcal during a buffet lunch, whereas following a high-fiber cereal (Fiber One)™ they ate 798 kcal during lunch. If the energy intake of breakfast was included in the calculation, the high fiber group ate about 192 fewer kcal. Cybulski et al.[18] reported that when crackers supplemented with psyllium were given as a preload food intake decreased during the test meal. In contrast, Burley et al.[16] did not see any effect of high-fiber breakfasts, containing guar gum and wheat bran-supplemented foods, on lunchtime intake. Most evidence indicates that intake of a high-fiber meal may be satiating, that is, it may decrease the length of a meal. Furthermore, it may decrease intake at the next meal.

## III. LONG-TERM FIBER TRIALS

Short-term effects on food intake are not of great interest to those attempting to lose weight or those interested in maintaining their goal body weight after weight loss. Most of the studies in the fiber/weight loss literature address the effects of fiber on body weight regulation during relatively long time periods. Twenty-six[10,24-41] of the 38 individual trials that evaluated the effect of fiber on body weight found a decrease in body weight following a high-fiber regimen. Unfortunately, in many of these studies the effects on body weight were small. Also, a large number of the studies were not double blinded and some even failed to include a placebo control. Those that included placebo controls did not always control for the energy value of the placebo compared to that of the fiber supplement.[32,33] Even a small energy difference between the low- and high-fiber supplement can affect body weight in a long-term study. For example, a 60 kcal difference per day could theoretically result in a 3 lb difference over a 6-month period.

Only a few of the studies in the literature have been carefully controlled and still one finds significant problems in the design or the conclusions of such studies. For example, Rossner and colleagues evaluated the effects of a cereal and citrus fruit fiber supplement on body weight in obese subjects who were participants in a slimming club.[32] In 1985, these investigators published a paper in "Dietary Fiber and Obesity", in which they studied 60 female patients. These subjects were instructed to follow a low calorie diet containing about 1400 kcal per day. In addition, the subjects ingested six tablets (fiber or placebo) three times a day with 300 ml of water 20 to 30 min before meals. Ingestion of all of the fiber tablets (270 mg each) would lead to an additional 5 g of dietary fiber per day. The energy content of each tablet was 1 kcal. The placebo tablets contained corn starch and saccharum and contained about 3 kcal. Thus, the fiber tablets contributed 18 kcal/day and the placebo tablets 54 kcal/day. After 8 weeks on the study, no differences were noted in food intake or in hunger ratings; both groups ingested on average less than 1200 kcal. The authors also stated than no differences were observed in body weight between the groups. In 1987 the same authors published another manuscript describing the effect of two different fiber supplements on body weight and food intake.[33] They once again evaluated overweight women who were instructed to eat a low calorie diet. In Study I they evaluated the effect of 5 g/day of a dietary fiber supplement and in Study II they studied the effect of 7 g/day of a dietary fiber supplement on body weight. Study I was conducted for 8 weeks, whereas Study II was conducted for 12 weeks. In Study I the high-fiber group lost 1 kg more weight than the control group and in Study II, the high-fiber group lost 2.1 kg more than the low-fiber group. There is a remarkable resemblance between Study I of this publication and the Rossner paper published in 1985.[32] In fact, the energy intakes of the subjects in these studies are identical at all time points. In 1985, Rossner et al. stated that there were no significant difference in weight loss between the two groups, but in 1987 concluded that the 1 kg difference was significant. It appears that they used a different means of analyzing their data. In any event, a 1 kg difference in weight loss is not necessary meaningful to the patient participating in a 2-month weight loss program. At least 7 g of a dietary supplement seems to be necessarily for a meaningful small effect in a group of overweight women on a weight loss program. A number of other reports, not always placebo controlled or double blind, have suggested a minor benefit in weight loss when a fiber supplement is used.[34-36] In none of these studies is there a major effect of the fiber supplement on body weight.

As in the acute studies, a number of the long-term studies found that food intake or hunger were decreased in the high fiber groups.[19,23,26,30,31,35,42-48] In most studies only qualitative measures of hunger were made. This can be a problem since results from a questionnaire about hunger may not agree with actual food intake data.[21] In studies in which food intake was measured the effects of fiber on food intake were not potent. Also, there are problems in interpreting such results, since quantitation of food intake is extremely difficult. Stevens et al.[48] carefully evaluated food intake by providing all of the food for the subjects for a 14-day period. They found no effect of fiber on digestible energy intake. However, many other variables aside from fiber intake might affect food intake. Stevens et al.[48] used covariate analysis to control for conditions that might have altered food intake including menses, menstrual cramps, medications, colds, and meals delivered outside the research unit. When these data were corrected for the latter conditions, the subjects ingesting the psyllium or psyllium plus bran-supplemented crackers ingested 115 to 157 fewer kcal/day than the control group. There was no effect of wheat bran alone on food intake. Almost all of those studies using fiber supplements in the form of pills failed to note any effect on energy intake.

## IV. EFFECT OF DIETARY FIBER ON NUTRIENT DIGESTIBILITY AND ABSORPTION

A study by Rigaud et al.[49] suggests that small effects of dietary fiber supplements on body weight may be due to fecal energy losses. These authors evaluated the effect of a fiber supplement (similar to those used in the above studies) on fecal output in 10 female and 10 male normal volunteers. The energy content of the stool samples was evaluated by bomb calorimetry. The fiber-treated subjects excreted 173 kcal/day, whereas the placebo-treated subjects excreted 153 kcal/day. Although the subjects on the high-fiber diet demonstrated a decrease in hunger rating compared with the placebo group, no differences in food intake were noted during this 4-week study. The differences in fecal output may not be of biological significance. The increased energy present in fecal samples of the high-fiber group was most likely due to malabsorption of the dietary fiber. Since little of the energy from the fermented dietary fiber is biologically available to the subject, they have not actually lost a major source of energy. If, however, the loss of dietary fiber "carries" along macronutrients that would normally be absorbed, this effect could be significant. This seems unlikely, since the 7.3 g of dietary fiber could account for the

20 kcal difference in fecal energy output each day, if one assumes that most of the fiber is carbohydrate. Stevens et al.[48] found that ingestion of fiber-supplemented crackers resulted in an increase in fecal energy output. The increase in fecal energy was less than the energy increase in the crackers derived from the addition of fiber. In another study, a high-fiber diet did appear to result in an increase in fecal fat excretion, which might result in a meaningful loss of energy.[50]

Fiber is not absorbed and reaches the colon where it can be fermented by the colonic microflora. This might result in gas production and a feeling or bloating or abdominal pain, which could result in a decrease in food intake or an altered perception of hunger. Stevens et al.[48] reported that psyllium of psyllium plus wheat bran-supplemented crackers increased bloating and flatulence in patients. However, this effect seemed to be unrelated to food intake, as evaluated by analysis of covariance. We[21] evaluated the correlation between colonic fermentation of fiber and food intake by measuring breath hydrogen, a product of bacterial fermentation. Ingestion of high-fiber cereals resulted in a greater excretion of breath hydrogen than ingestion of low-fiber cereals. However, there was not a perfect correlation. For example, Shredded Wheat intake increased gas production twice as much as ingestion of Post Toasties, but failed to alter food intake. All Bran and Fiber One, which decreased food intake, resulted in the highest levels of breath hydrogen.

## V. CONCLUSIONS

Depending on one's bias the above data could suggest that fiber alters food intake and body weight (Table 2). However, one cannot recommend fiber supplements as a means to control weight or lose weight at the current time with any degree of security. Few studies have been conducted for longer than a 1 month period in subjects who have not been on a weight reduction plan. Data in obese subjects need to be collected in a controlled fashion using a variety of sources of fiber during periods of weight loss and weight maintenance. Many studies are confounded by the reduction in calories consumed resulting from dietary consultation. If the subjects are eating only 1200 kcal/day it is difficult to evaluate whether dietary fiber further reduces intake. It might be better to study obese subjects who simply add high-fiber food to their diet. This would result in a low-fat diet, which might also decrease the incidence of cancer and heart disease. A study by Kendall et al.[51] suggests that such low-fat and high-fiber foods may help patients lose weight. Simply adding fiber, through pills or powders, to a high-fat diet probably will not be a useful approach in the management of weight loss.

**TABLE 2**
**Variability in Fiber Studies (Design and Responses)**

| | |
|---|---|
| Subject numbers | 7 to 122 |
| Length of studies | 1 meal to 56 weeks |
| Fiber types | High-fiber foods: fruits and vegetables<br>Fiber isolates: wheat bran, oat bran, guar gum, psyllium, methylcellulose, cellulose, citrus fruit fiber, kaolin, glucomannon |
| Dose range | 1 g methylcellulose to 50 g/day of high-fiber foods |
| Design | Open, blind, and double blind<br>No placebo and placebo controlled<br>Parallel and cross-over |
| Measurement of hunger and satiety | Visual analog scales, dietary recall, quantification of ingested food |
| Response range | Acute studies: from no effect on food intake to a decrease of 590 kcal/day deficit<br>Chronic trials: from no effect on body weight to a 2.5 kg difference in weight loss between high-fiber vs. low-fiber groups |

## REFERENCES


1. Council on Scientific Affairs, Dietary fiber and health, *J. Am. Med. Assoc.,* 262, 542, 1989.
2. Trowell, H., Definitions of fiber, *Lancet,* 1, 503, 1974.
3. Haber, G. B., Heaton, K. W., Murphy, B., and Burroughs, L., Depletion and disruption of dietary fibre. Effects on satiety, plasma-glucose and serum-insulin, *Lancet,* 2, 679, 1977.
4. Holt, S., Heading, R. C., Carter, D. C., Prescott, L. F., and Tothill, P., Effect of gel fibre on gastric emptying and absorption of glucose and paracetabol, *Lancet,* 1, 636, 1979.
5. Farrell, D. J., Girle, L., and Arthur, J., Effects of dietary fibre on the apparent digestibility of major food components and on blood lipids in men, *Aust. J. Exp. Biol. Med. Sci.,* 56, 469, 1978.
6. Kelsay, J. L., Behall, K. M., and Prather, E. S., Effect of fiber from fruits and vegetables on metabolic responses of human subjects. I. Bowel transit time, number of defecations, fecal weight, urinary excretions of energy and nitrogen and apparent digestibilities of energy, nitrogen and fat, *Am. J. Clin. Nutr.,* 31, 1149, 1978.
7. Stevens, J., Does dietary fiber affect food intake and body weight?, *J. Am. Diet. Assoc.,* 88, 939, 1988.

8. Blundell, J. E., and Burley, V. J., Satiation, satiety and the action of fibre on food intake, *Int. J. Obes.,* 11 (Suppl. 1), 9, 1987.
9. Burley, V. J., and Blundell, J. E., Action of Dietary fiber on the satiety cascade. In: *Dietary Fiber: Chemistry, Physiology & Health Effects,* D. Kritchevsky, C. Bonfield, and J. W. Anderson, Eds. Plenum Press, New York, 1990, 227.
10. Pilch, S. M., Ed., Physiological effects and health consequences of dietary fiber. Life Sciences Research Office. Federation of American Societies for Experimental Biology, Bethesda, 1987.
11. Yudkin, J., The causes and cure of obesity, *Lancet,* 2, 1135, 1959.
12. Barkeling, B., Ryttig, K., and Rossner, S., Objective analysis of human eating behaviour and food preferences, *1st Eur. Congr. Obes.,* 136, 1988.
13. Bolton, R. P., Heaton, K. W., and Burroughs, L. F., The role of dietary fibre on satiety, glucose, and insulin: studies with fruit and fruit juice, *Am. J. Clin. Nutr.,* 34, 211, 1981.
14. Bryson, E., Dore, C., and Garrow, J. S., Wholemeal bread and satiety, *J. Hum. Nutr.,* 34, 113, 1980.
15. Burley, V. J., Leeds, A. R., and Blundell, J. E., The effect of high and low-fibre breakfasts on hunger, satiety and food intake in a subsequent meal, *Int. J. Obes.,* 11 (Suppl. 1), 87, 1987.
16. Burley, V. J., Leeds, A. R., and Blundell, J. E., The effect of high and low fiber breakfasts on hunger, satiety, and food intake in a subsequent meal, *Int. J. Obes.,* (Suppl. 1), 87, 1987.
17. Cocchi, M., Siniscalchi, C., Billi, G. C., Sciarretta, G., DeMuti, R., and Ruffilli, E., Alimentary fibre effect on feeding of satiety: subjective evaluation and biochemical data modifications, *Giorn. Clin. Med.,* 65, 99, 1984.
18. Cybulski, K. A., Lachausslee, J., and Kissileff, H. R., The threshold for satiating effectiveness of psyllium in a nutrient base, *Physiol. Behav.,* 51, 89, 1992.
19. Ellis, P. R., Apling, E. C., Leeds, A. R., Peterson, D. B., and Jepson, E. W., Guar bread and satiety: effects of an acceptable new product in overweight diabetic patients and normal subjects, *J. Plant Foods,* 6, 253, 1985.
20. Grimes, D. S., and Gordon, C., Satiety value of wholemeal and white bread, *Lancet,* 2, 106, 1978.
21. Levine, A. S., Tallman, J. R., Grace, M. K., Parker, S. A., Billington, C. J., and Levitt, M. D., Effect of breakfast cereals on short-term food intake, *Am. J. Clin. Nutr.,* 50, 1303, 1989.
22. Porikos, K., and Hagamen, S., Is fiber satiating? Effects of a high fiber preload on subsequent food intake of normal-weight and obese young men, *Appetite,* 7, 153, 1986.
23. Wilmshurst, P., and Crawley, J. C. W., The measurement of gastric transit time in obese subjects using 24Na and the effects of energy content and guar gum on gastric emptying, *Br. J. Nutr.,* 44, 1, 1980.
24. Dodson, P. M., Stocks, J., Holdsworth, G., and Galton, D. J., High-fibre and low-fat diets in diabetes mellitus, *Br. J. Nutr.,* 46, 289, 1981.
25. Ehmann, D., and Ressin, W., About the significance of dietary fiber in the dietetic treatment of overweight individuals, *Pharm. Ztg.,* 130, 124, 1985.

26. Evans, E., and Miller, D. S., Bulking agents in the treatment of obesity, *Nutr. Metabol.,* 18, 199, 1975.
27. Frati-Munari, A. C., Fernandez-Harp, J. A., Becerril, M., Chavez-Negrete, A., and Banales-Ham, M., Decrease in serum lipids, glycemia and body weight by Plantago psyllium in obese and diabetic patients, *Arch. Invest. Med.,* 14, 259, 1983.
28. Geliebler, A. A., The effects of equal caloric loads of protein, fat and carbohydrate and noncaloric loads on food intake in the rat and man, Ph.D. thesis, 1976.
29. Krotkiewski, M., Effect of guar gum on body-weight, hunger ratings and metabolism in obese subjects, *Br. J. Nutr.,* 52, 97, 1984.
30. Krotkiewski, M., Use of fibres in different weight reduction programs, in *Current Topics in Nutrition and Disease. Vol. 14. Dietary Fiber and Obesity,* P. Bjoerntorp, G. V. Vahoung, and D. Kritchevsky, Eds. (New York: Alan R. Liss, Inc., 1985), pp. 85-109.
31. Mickelson, O., Makdani, D. D., Cotton, R. H., Titcomb, S. T., Colney, J. C., and Gatty, R., Effects on a high fibre diet on weight loss in college-age males, *Am. J. Clin. Nutr.,* 32, 1703, 1979.
32. Rossner, S., Zweigbergk, D., and Ohlin, A., Effects of dietary fibre in treatment of over weight out-patients, in *Dietary Fiber and Obesity,* P. Bjoerntorp, G. V. Vahoung, and D. Kritchevsky, Eds. (New York: Alan R. Liss, Inc., 1985), pp. 69-76.
33. Rossner, S., Von Zweigbergk, D., Ohlin, A., and Ryttig, K. R., Weight reduction with dietary fibre supplements. Results of two double-blind studies, *Acta. Med. Scand.,* 222(1), 83, 1987.
34. Ryttig, K. R., Larson, S., and Haegh, L., Behandling av lett til moderat overveldige personer, *Tidddkr Nor. Laegeforen,* 104, 989, 1984.
35. Ryttig, K. R., Larsen, S., and Haegh, L., Treatment of slightly to moderately overweight persons. A double-blind placebo-controlled investigation with diet and fiber tablets (Dumo Vital), in *Dietary Fiber and Obesity,* P. Bjoerntorp, G. V. Vahoung, and D. Kritchevsky, Eds. (New York: Alan R. Liss, Inc., 1985), pp. 77-84.
36. Solum, T. T., Fiber tablets, DumoVital — an aid to start weight reduction [Nor], *Tidsskrift Nor. Laegeforen.,* 103, 1707, 1983.
37. Stevens, J., VanSoest, P. J., Robertson, J. B., and Levitsky, D. A., The use of multicolored plastic pellets to measure mean transit time by analysis of a single stool, *Am. J. Clin. Nutr.,* 46, 1048, 1987.
38. Valle-Jones, J. C., The evaluation of a new appetite-reducing agent (Prefil) in the management of obesity, *Br. J. Clin. Prac.,* 34, 72, 1980.
39. Weinreich, J., Pederson, O., and Denison, K., Role of bran in normals: serum levels of cholesterol, triglyceride, calcium and total 3 alphahydroxycholanic acid, and intestinal transit time, *Acta. Med. Scand.,* 202, 125, 1977.
40. Weinsier, R. L., Johnston, M. H., Doleys, D. M., and Bacon, J. A., Dietary management of obesity: evaluation of the time-energy displacement diet in terms of its efficacy and nutritional adequacy for long-term weight control, *Br. J. Nutr.,* 47, 367, 1982.

41. Weinsier, R. L., Bacon, J. A., and Birch, R., Time-calorie displacement diet for weight control: a prospective evaluation of its adequacy for maintaining normal nutritional status, *Int. J. Obes.*, 7, 539, 1983.
42. Duncan, K. H., Bacon, J. A., and Weinsier, R. L., The effects of high and low energy density diets on satiety, energy intake, and eating time of obese and nonobese subjects, *Am. J. Clin. Nutr.*, 37, 763, 1983.
43. Hylander, B., and Rossner, S., Effects of dietary fiber intake before meals on weight loss and hunger in a weight-reducing club, *Acta Med. Scand.*, 213, 217, 1983.
44. Anonymous. What should lipid-lowering nutrition include? [German], *Fortschritte Med.*, 106 (Suppl. 46), 19, 1988.
45. Pitto, G., Sganga, F., and Mereta, F., Una nuova fibra vegetale. Studio clinico condotto su 20 soggetti voluntari sani, Minerva Dietol, *Gastroenterology*, 33, 235, 1987.
46. Quaade, F., Vrist, E., and Astrup, A., Fibre supplementation to very low calorie diet normalises hunger and alleviates constipation, *1st Eur. Congr. Obes.*, 289, 1988.
47. Shearer, R., Effects of bulk-producing tablets on hunger intensity in dieting patients, *Curr. Ther. Res.*, 19, 433, 1976.
48. Stevens, J., Levitsky, D. A., VanSoest, P. J., Robertson, J. B., Kalkwarf, H. J., and Roe, D. A., Effect of psyllium gum and wheat bran on spontaneous energy intake, *Am. J. Clin. Nutr.*, 46, 812, 1987.
49. Rigaud, D., Ryttig, K. R., Leeds, A. R., Bard, D., and Apfelbaum, M., Effects of a moderate dietary fibre supplement on hunger rating, energy input and faecal energy output in young, healthy volunteers; a randomized, double-blind cross-over trial, *Int. J. Obes.*, (Suppl. 1), 73, 1987.
50. Levine, A. S., and Silvis, S. E., Absorption of whole peanuts, peanut oil, and peanut butter, *N. Engl. J. Med.*, 303, 917, 1980.
51. Kendall, A., Levitsky, D. A., Strupp, B. J., and Lissner, L., Weight loss on a low-fat diet: consequence of the imprecision of the control of food intake on humans, *Am. J. Clin. Nutr.*, 53(5), 1124, 1991.

# Index

## D



## E

F



G

## H



## I



## K



## L

## T

**V**



**W**